External Ear Disease

Editors

MATTHEW B. HANSON
ESTHER X. VIVAS

OTOLARYNGOLOGIC CLINICS OF NORTH AMERICA

www.oto.theclinics.com

Consulting Editor
SUJANA S. CHANDRASEKHAR

October 2023 • Volume 56 • Number 5

ELSEVIER

1600 John F. Kennedy Boulevard • Suite 1800 • Philadelphia, Pennsylvania, 19103-2899

http://www.oto.theclinics.com

OTOLARYNGOLOGIC CLINICS OF NORTH AMERICA Volume 56, Number 5
October 2023 ISSN 0030-6665, ISBN-13: 978-0-443-13033-5

Editor: Stacy Eastman
Developmental Editor: Malvika Shah

Otolaryngologic Clinics of North America (ISSN 0030-6665) is published bimonthly by Elsevier, Inc., 360 Park Avenue South, New York, NY 10010-1710. Months of issue are February, April, June, August, October, and December. Business and Editorial Offices: 1600 John F. Kennedy Blvd., Suite 1800, Philadelphia, PA 19103-2899. Customer Service Office: 6277 Sea Harbor Drive, Orlando, FL 32887-4800. Periodicals postage paid at New York, NY and additional mailing offices. Subscription prices are $468.00 per year (US individuals), $1117.00 per year (US institutions), $100.00 per year (US & Canadian student/resident), $599.00 per year (Canadian individuals), $1416.00 per year (Canadian institutions), $653.00 per year (international individuals), $1416.00 per year (international institutions), $270.00 per year (international student/resident). Foreign air speed delivery is included in all *Clinics'* subscription prices. All prices are subject to change without notice. **POSTMASTER:** Send address changes to *Otolaryngologic Clinics of North America*, Elsevier Health Sciences Division, Subscription Customer Service, 3251 Riverport Lane, Maryland Heights, MO 63043. **Telephone: 1-800-654-2452 (U.S. and Canada); 314-447-8871 (outside U.S. and Canada). Fax: 314-447-8029. E-mail: journalscustomerservice-usa@elsevier.com (for print support); journalsonlinesupport-usa@elsevier.com (for online support).**

Reprints. For copies of 100 or more of articles in this publication, please contact the Commercial Reprints Department, Elsevier Inc., 360 Park Avenue South, New York, NY 10010-1710. Tel.: 212-633-3874; Fax: 212-633-3820; E-mail: reprints@elsevier.com.

Otolaryngologic Clinics of North America is also published in Spanish by McGraw-Hill Interamericana Editores S.A., P.O. Box 5-237, 06500 Mexico D.F., Mexico.

Otolaryngologic Clinics of North America is covered in *MEDLINE/PubMed (Index Medicus), Current Contents/Clinical Medicine, Excerpta Medica, BIOSIS, Science Citation Index,* and *ISI/BIOMED.*

Contributors

CONSULTING EDITOR

SUJANA S. CHANDRASEKHAR, MD, FACS, FAAOHNS
Consulting Editor, Otolaryngologic Clinics of North America, President, American Otological Society, Past President, American Academy of Otolaryngology-Head and Neck Surgery, Partner, ENT & Allergy Associates, LLP, Clinical Professor, Department of Otolaryngology-Head and Neck Surgery, Zucker School of Medicine at Hofstra/Northwell, Clinical Associate Professor, Department of Otolaryngology-Head and Neck Surgery, Icahn School of Medicine at Mount Sinai, New York, New York

EDITORS

MATTHEW B. HANSON, MD
Director of Otology and Neurotology, Department of Otolaryngology, SUNY, Assistant Professor, SUNY Downstate College of Medicine, Chief of Otology at UHB and KCHC, Director of Service, Otolaryngology, Kings County Hospital Center, Brooklyn, New York

ESTHER X. VIVAS, MD
Division Chief of Otology and Neurotology, Director, Surgical Dissection Laboratory, and Temporal Bone Course, Professor, Department of Otolaryngology–Head and Neck Surgery Otology-Neurotology, Emory University, Atlanta, Georgia

AUTHORS

MATTHEW ADAMS, MD
Resident Physician, SUNY Downstate, Brooklyn, New York

JENNIFER ALYONO, MD, MS
Clinical Assistant Professor, Department of Otolaryngology–Head and Neck Surgery, Stanford University School of Medicine, Palo Alto, California

VALERIANNA AMOROSA, MD
Professor, Corporal Michael J. Crescenz VA Medical Center, Philadelphia, Pennsylvania

KATHERINE BELDEN, MD
Division of Infectious Diseases, Thomas Jefferson University Hospital, Philadelphia, Pennsylvania

TRAVIS W. BLALOCK, MD
Associate Professor, Department of Dermatology, Emory University School of Medicine, Atlanta, Georgia

KAITLYN A. BROOKS, MD
Department of Otolaryngology–Head and Neck Surgery, Emory University, Atlanta, Georgia

JUSTIN T. CHEELEY, MD
Assistant Professor, Department of Dermatology, Emory University School of Medicine, Atlanta, Georgia

STEVEN D. CURRY, MD
Department of Otolaryngology–Head and Neck Surgery, University of Nebraska Medical Center, Omaha, Nebraska

PAYAM ENTEZAMI, MD
Resident, Department of Otolaryngology–Head Neck Surgery, Louisiana State University Health, Shreveport, Louisiana

PAUL W. GIDLEY, MD, FACS
Department of Head and Neck Surgery, The University of Texas MD Anderson Cancer Center, Houston, Texas

JENNIFER H. GROSS, MD
Assistant Professor of Otolaryngology–Head and Neck Surgery, Emory University, Winship Cancer Institute, Atlanta, Georgia

MICKIE HAMITER, MD
Department of Otolaryngology, Columbia University Irving Medical Center, New York, New York

MATTHEW B. HANSON, MD
Director of Otology and Neurotology, Department of Otolaryngology, SUNY, Assistant Professor, SUNY Downstate College of Medicine, Chief of Otology at UHB and KCHC, Director of Service, Otolaryngology, Kings County Hospital Center, Brooklyn, New York

LATRICE M. HOGUE, MD
Department of Dermatology, Emory University School of Medicine, Atlanta, Georgia

JACOB B. HUNTER, MD
Associate Professor, Otology/Neurotology, Division Chief, Department of Otolaryngology–Head and Neck Surgery, Thomas Jefferson University Hospital, Philadelphia, Pennsylvania

BRADLEY KESSER, MD
Professor and Vice Chair, Department of Otolaryngology–Head and Neck Surgery, University of Virginia School of Medicine, University of Virginia Department of Otolaryngology, Charlottesville, Virginia

ANA H. KIM, MD
Department of Otolaryngology, Columbia University Irving Medical Center, New York, New York

JENNA E. KOBLINSKI, MD
Dermatology Resident, Department of Dermatology, Emory University School of Medicine, Atlanta, Georgia

PETER J. KULLAR, MA, PhD, FRCS
Clinical Instructor, Department of Otolaryngology–Head and Neck Surgery, Stanford University School of Medicine, Palo Alto, California

REBECCA LEIBOWITZ, BS
Emory University School of Medicine, Atlanta, Georgia

FRANK E. LUCENTE, MD
Professor and Former Chairman, Department of Otolaryngology, SUNY Downstate Medical Center, Brooklyn, New York

GAURI MANKEKAR, MD, PhD
Assistant Professor, Department of Otolaryngology–Head Neck Surgery, Louisiana State University Health, Shreveport, Louisiana

ANNE K. MAXWELL, MD
Department of Otolaryngology–Head and Neck Surgery, University of Nebraska Medical Center, Omaha, Nebraska

ERIKA MCCARTY WALSH, MD
Department of Otolaryngology–Head and Neck Surgery, The University of Alabama at Birmingham, Birmingham, Alabama

SUYASH MOHAN, MD
Department of Radiology, University of Pennsylvania Perelman School of Medicine, Philadelphia, Pennsylvania

DANIEL MORRISON, MD
Department of Otolaryngology–Head and Neck Surgery, University of Virginia School of Medicine, University of Virginia Department of Otolaryngology, Charlottesville, Virginia

TINA MUNJAL, MD
Department of Otolaryngology–Head and Neck Surgery, Stanford University School of Medicine, Palo Alto, California

BRIAN PERRY, MD
Department of Otolaryngology–Head and Neck Surgery, UT Health San Antonio, Joe R. and Teresa Lozano Long School of Medicine, San Antonio, Texas

ANN WOODHOUSE PLUM, MD
Department of Otolaryngology, State of New York Downstate Medical Center, Brooklyn, New York

MALLORY RAYMOND, MD
Assistant Professor, Department of Otolaryngology–Head and Neck Surgery, Mayo Clinic, Jacksonville, Florida

DONALD TAN, MD
Department of Otolaryngology–Head and Neck Surgery, The University of Texas Southwestern Medical Center, Dallas, Texas

MICHELE WONG, MD
Department of Otolaryngology, State of New York Downstate Medical Center, Brooklyn New York

Contents

This article provides a historical overview of disorders of the external ear, focusing on advances in technology, pharmacology, and education that have been beneficial. While the diagnosis and treatment of various conditions involving the external ear canal and auricle continue to evolve, it remains to be seen how the latest challenges will be met.

The external auditory canal is a highly specialized skin appendage whose primary purpose is to provide a pathway for the transmission of sound to the tympanic membrane and beyond. It is also a frequent source of symptoms for our patients. Sources of pain, hearing loss, tinnitus, itching, and other sensations can be inferred from an appropriate history. This should be followed by a thorough cleaning of the ear, so that a thorough examination can be performed.

The external canal is a unique environment that has an elaborate mechanism for self-cleaning and protection. The fundamental basis of this is the epithelial migration of the desquamating layers of the keratinizing epithelium that lines the entire canal and ear drum. This migratory movement results in a "conveyor belt" effect where the dead skin is moved out of the bony ear canal to the cartilaginous portion, where it is lifted off with the help of glandular skin secretions and the hairs of the canal to form what we call "ear wax." The ear wax has numerous protective properties and is essential to the health of the external ear. The protective properties are due to chemical properties of the wax, in addition to intrinsic chemical secretions by the sebaceous and cerumen apocrine glands. The protection also comes from a diverse population of organisms that exist in the external ear that are usually saprophytic, commensal, and symbiotic, but in some cases, they can become parasitic and pathologic. Detection and quantification of the members of this biome has been difficult, and their overall role in the normal biome of the ear and their transition into pathogens remain an area of active research and investigation.

a high index of suspicion for fungal causes of ear canal disease is critical. Fungal pathogens may be an especially important cause of ear canal disease in certain populations, including patients with diabetes, patients recently treated with antibiotics, and immunosuppressed patients. Opportunistic fungal infections of the ear canal are an emerging concern.

Acquired stenosis of the external ear canal (ASEEC) is a relatively uncommon condition. Stenosis or narrowing of the external ear canal (EEC) occurs lateral to the tympanic membrane resulting in a skin lined blind canal. Recurrent otorrhea, and conductive hearing loss are typical clinical features. Although ASEEC can be due to different etiologies, a common pathogenesis, namely an inflammatory cascade, has been implicated. Clinical evaluation, audiogram, and Computed tomography (CT scan) form the mainstay of diagnosis. Surgery is the primary modality for treatment. Restenosis is the most common postsurgical complication.

Congenital anomalies of the external auditory canal (EAC) are classically divided into congenital aural atresia (CAA) and congenital aural stenosis (CAS). CAA can present as an isolated anomaly, unilateral or bilateral, or in the setting of a craniofacial syndrome. Hearing testing (ABR with air and bone conduction thresholds for both ears) early in the perinatal period is important to document hearing thresholds. Hearing status thus informs parent counseling on options for hearing habilitation: Bone conducting technology is a must for children with bilateral CAA to support normal speech and language development. Bone conducting technology should be considered for children with unilateral CAA; benefits are unclear. In select candidates, atresia repair can provide improved hearing with a clean, dry, epithelialized ear canal. First branchial cleft cyst or sinus is rare; high index of suspicion is needed to diagnose along with high-resolution CT. Congenital aural stenosis (CAS) is a rare condition, and hearing testing should be similar to that in children with CAA. Early (age 4–5) CT imaging is recommended in the setting of a canal <2 mm or pinpoint canal to evaluate for trapped skin/ear canal cholesteatoma.

Cutaneous diseases of the ear encompass a wide range of symptoms, complaints, and factors that negatively impact patients' well-being. These observations are frequently encountered by otolaryngologists and other physicians who treat individuals with ear-related issues. In this document, we aim to offer up-to-date information on diagnosing, predicting outcomes, and treating commonly occurring ear diseases.

Primary EAC neoplasms include benign and malignant lesions of bony, glandular or cutaneous origin. Small, benign slow growing bony neoplasms are often asymptomatic, diagnosed incidentally and might not require intervention. Both malignant and benign neoplasms of cutaneous and glandular origin can present with symptoms of chronic otitis externa, leading to delays in diagnosis. Prompt biopsy of soft tissue lesions associated with non-resolving otitis externa are warranted. Local and regional imaging is helpful to understand disease extent and origin, but even early-stage malignant neoplasms require aggressive surgical treatment.

Acute radiotherapy (RT)-induced external ear soft tissue changes start with erythema and dry desquamation and may progress to moist desquamation and epidermal ulceration. Chronic RT-induced changes include epithelial atrophy and subcutaneous fibrosis. Although RT-induced radiation dermatitis has been well studied, interventions for soft tissue disease involving the external auditory canal (EAC) warrant investigation. Medical management includes topical steroid treatment for EAC radiation dermatitis and topical antibiotic therapy for suppurative otitis externa. Hyperbaric oxygen and pentoxifylline–vitamin E therapy have shown promise for other applications, but their clinical effect on soft tissue EAC disease is currently undefined.

SBO is a life-threatening disease that requires a high index of suspicion based on these patients complex underlying medical co-morbidities and clinician's acumen. Once a diagnosis is made, is it critical to communicate and work closely with other multidisciplinary teams (neuroradiology for appropriate choice of imaging study and interpretation; infectious disease for appropriate medical treatment and duration; internist to properly manage their underlying medical co-morbidities). Despite advances in imaging, the diagnosis is first made based on clinical judgment, appropriate culture, and tissue biopsy.

OTOLARYNGOLOGIC CLINICS OF NORTH AMERICA

SERIES OF RELATED INTEREST

Facial Plastic Surgery Clinics
Available at: https://www.facialplastic.theclinics.com/

THE CLINICS ARE AVAILABLE ONLINE!
Access your subscription at:
www.theclinics.com

Foreword

The External Auditory Canal Should Not Be, but Is, Often Overlooked

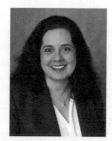

Sujana S. Chandrasekhar, MD, FACS, FAAOHNS
Consulting Editor

Discussions about the ear usually focus on the pinna and jump to the tympanic membrane (TM) and middle and inner ear, traversing but ignoring the external auditory canal (EAC), similar to the way that sound waves traverse the ear canal to reach the TM. However, disorders of the EAC, which is also referred to as the external auditory meatus or EAM, affect a significant percentage of the population of all ages, resulting in great physical, monetary, and even emotional costs. A majority of pathologic conditions affecting the EAC require office-based and medical treatment; only a small minority will need surgical intervention. As surgeons, the more "mundane" care of ear canal issues may not seem compelling, but the importance of this treatment is obvious in our patients' gratitude.

Acute otitis externa (AOE) affects at least 1 in 123 people in the United States, with a predictable seasonal predilection in warmer weather with water exposure, and a nearly equal split between children and adults.[1] Other data show that approximately 10% of people will develop otitis externa (OE) in their lifetime, with 95% of cases being AOE and 5% being chronic otitis externa (COE).[2] COE can be related to one of several dermatologic aberrations and causative pathogens. For inflammatory disorders of the EAC, various otic drops, lotions, creams, oils, and powders have been used with varying degrees of success. Knowledge of the options and when to offer them is crucial.

External ear canal cholesteatomas and keratosis obturans are both rare conditions of the EAC that are often mistaken for each other clinically but require quite different approaches. Similarly, osteomas and exostoses, both bony growths of the EAC, are also not interchangeable, and when they demand intervention, approaches are likewise different. Congenital aural atresia occurs in 1:10,000 to 1:20,000 live births. Its

Otolaryngol Clin N Am 56 (2023) xiii–xv
https://doi.org/10.1016/j.otc.2023.06.014
0030-6665/23/© 2023 Published by Elsevier Inc.

oto.theclinics.com

management is highly nuanced and has changed over time with the advent of osseointegrated implants that can provide excellent hearing benefit.

The EAC is lined with specialized epithelium that is different in the outer third (cartilaginous portion) of the canal compared with the inner two-thirds of the canal, which is bony. The skin of the cartilaginous canal is thickened with a spongy subcutaneous layer possessing modified sebaceous glands called cerumen glands; the skin of the bony canal is thin and flush against the canal wall bone and does not possess ceruminous glands or hair follicles.[3] Ear wax, or cerumen, is produced by the cerumen glands of the cartilaginous EAC and is a natural lubricant, which may also possess some antimicrobial properties. Whether a person's cerumen is wet or dry is determined by one single-nucleotide polymorphism of a single gene (ABCC11); individuals with dry wax, especially if they also use hearing aids, may suffer from cerumen impaction at higher frequency.[4] The management of cerumen, considered so commonplace among otolaryngologists, has resulted in the most widely read Clinical Practice Guideline and Update from the American Academy of Otolaryngology–Head and Neck Surgery.[5] We should not forget about necrotizing or "malignant" OE, its pathogens and treatment, or actual malignant neoplasms—squamous cell carcinoma, basal cell carcinoma, melanoma, ceruminoma—that arise in the EAC. Damage to the EAC can result from automanipulation by the patient as well as from radiation exposure for other tumors.

Drs Esther X. Vivas and Matthew Hanson have put together an outstanding series of articles in this issue of Otolaryngologic Clinics of North America that covers the various pathologic conditions listed above and more and how to assess and manage patients who present with these problems. Having read all of the articles, including a wonderful preface by Dr Frank Lucente highlighting the history of EAC care, you, the reader, will be well-equipped to manage the most recalcitrant of EAC conditions and will be well rewarded by a happy patient.

Sujana S. Chandrasekhar, MD, FACS, FAAOHNS
Consulting Editor
Otolaryngologic Clinics of North America
President, American Otological Society
Past President
American Academy of Otolaryngology–
Head and Neck Surgery
Partner, ENT and Allergy Associates, LLP
Co-Host, She's On Call
18 East 48th Street, 2nd Floor
New York, NY 10017, USA

E-mail address:
ssc@nyotology.com

REFERENCES

1. Centers for Disease Control and Prevention. Estimated burden of acute otitis externa—United States, 2003–2007. MMWR Morb Mortal Wkly Rep 2011;60(19):605–9.

2. Medina-Blasini Y, Sharman T. Otitis externa. In: StatPearls [Internet]. Treasure Island (FL): StatPearls Publishing; 2023. Available at: https://www.ncbi.nlm.nih.gov/books/NBK556055/. Accessed June 26, 2023.

3. Standrig S, Anand N, Birch R, et al. Gray's anatomy 40th edition. 41st edition. Amsterdam: Elsevier; 2016. p. 639–61.
4. Mozaffari M, Nash R, Tucker AS. Anatomy and development of the mammalian external auditory canal: implications for understanding canal disease and deformity. Front Cell Dev Biol 2021;8:1–11. https://doi.org/10.3389/fcell.2020.617354, 617354.
5. Schwartz SR, Magit AE, Rosenfeld RM, et al. Clinical practice guideline (update): earwax (cerumen impaction). Otolaryngol Head Neck Surg 2017;156(1_suppl): S1–29. https://doi.org/10.1177/0194599816671491 [Erratum appears in Otolaryngol Head Neck Surg 2017;157(3):539. PMID: 28045591].

Preface

The Joys of "External Otology"

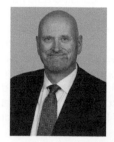 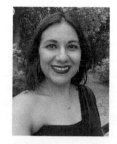

Matthew B. Hanson, MD   Esther X. Vivas, MD
Editors

The field of Otolaryngology–Head and Neck surgery covers far more than its label as a "specialty" implies. Our profession deals with all ages from infants to the aged and deals with problems as complex as skull base tumors, airway reconstruction in newborns, resection of large tumors of the head and neck, and reconstruction with microvascular tissue transfer. Indeed, the depth and breadth of this specialty are so daunting to many of our residents, they seek even further specialization through fellowships, often adding two or more years onto their training to become an "expert" in one area of our complex specialty. Having committed so much time in training for these sub-sub-subspecialties, we look forward to a career where we do battle with the most complex of problems. We do research to find how these problems arise and develop better ways to treat them. We publish our studies; we publicize our new techniques, and we embrace new technology and put ourselves out there as the "go-to expert" in our areas. We put out our shingle and wait for all these complex patients to come in for us to do our magic. When our first patient sits down in the chair and tells us they came to us because their ears are itchy, we roll our eyes and sigh.

Such is the nature of the external ear. It is the bastard child of otolaryngology. No one likes it, but we know that we own it, so we must tolerate it. Not one of us advertises ourselves as an "external otologist." None of us did a fellowship in the treatment of itchy ears. None of us seeks to see more patients with earwax impactions. None of us, when we are lying on our deathbed and are looking back on our lives, will think of all the "swimmer's ear" that we treated and feel confident we will be welcomed by Our Maker and be granted entry into paradise.

But the number of patients who seek treatment for ear canal issues is staggering. Problems such as earwax, ear itching, and insects in the ear are common, but often the "minor" complaints of ear fullness, hearing loss, ear itch, and ear pain can be the harbinger of a much more serious problem that can often be missed when these complaints are not appropriately investigated. Erroneous treatment of these ear

Otolaryngol Clin N Am 56 (2023) xvii–xviii
https://doi.org/10.1016/j.otc.2023.07.005
0030-6665/23/© 2023 Published by Elsevier Inc.

complaints in many primary care settings often complicates the problem. It is not uncommon to have patients referred that have undergone multiple courses of otic quinolone drops for ear pain due to TMJ issues. And now present with a florid yeast infection in the ear. A precipitous rise in infections caused by fungus and yeast is now occurring, especially in the Northeast United States, where emerging pathogens, such as *Candida auris*, are becoming increasingly prevalent and represent a considerable hazard in ICU settings.

When we were asked to coedit this issue, we made the decision to limit the subject matter to the external ear canal and not include subjects pertaining to the auricle, such as microtia and trauma. Even with this, we had difficulty in limiting the subject matter. Even with this limitation, we are aware that many subjects are not covered. More importantly, it was evident that many of the issues that we did cover have not had meaningful research performed in many years, and the articles contain few additional references from our current century. This is another example of how the diseases of the external canal are often overlooked or underappreciated.

We hope that we have produced a decent summary of the latest insights into many of the most common problems that are seen by the Otolaryngologist. Both of us are fellowship-trained Neurotologists, but this issue is targeted to all otolaryngologists and would be beneficial to many primary care practitioners as well. We want to thank Dr Sujana Chandrasekhar for her leadership and guidance in preparing this issue. We also thank the Editors and Staff at Elsevier Publishing, especially Stacy Eastman and Malvika Shah. Your patience with us was much appreciated. We hope the issue is a hit!

Matthew B. Hanson, MD
450 Clarkson Avenue
Box 126
Brooklyn, NY 11203, USA

Esther X. Vivas, MD
Department of Otolaryngology
550 Peachtree Street Northeast
MOT, Suite 1135
11th Floor
Atlanta, GA 30308, USA

E-mail addresses:
matthew.hanson@downstate.edu (M.B. Hanson)
evivas@emory.edu (E.X. Vivas)

Disorders of the External Ear-A Historical Perspective

Frank E. Lucente, MD

KEYWORDS

• External ear • Cerumen • Auricle • Otologic community

The external ear, namely the auricle and external auditory canal, have challenged physicians and other care givers since the dawn of humankind. The external ear has tremendous functional, and cosmetic, significance. It has been used as the site of ornamentation and social expression in various cultures over the centuries. It is also the most visible and accessible part of the delicate and complicated hearing process.

Certain anatomical and physical characteristics pose special challenges. The cartilage can vary tremendously in configuration. It has poor blood supply which makes treatment of infections which require blood-borne antibiotics difficult. The overlying perichondrium and skin can be used in the therapeutic process but the cartilage is a particular problem when it is damaged or infected.

The skin of the external ear can manifest generalized dermatoses. The skin and cartilage of the external ear can also be used in the reconstruction of damaged areas, such as the opposite auricle and the nose. Anatomical deformities of the auricle can be the source of much psychological distress.

Use of the auricle for ornamentation has been practiced for centuries. Certain tribal practices involve stretching the lobule and insertion of earrings or other decorative objects. With its adequate blood supply, this is generally well-tolerated. However, the recent practice of piercing the cartilage and inserting objects (sometimes as part of a weight-loss or smoking-cessation program) is less well-tolerated. The auricle can also be a site for the implementation of a form of acupuncture called auriculopuncture, especially in the Orient.

In 1957, Ben H. Senturia, an otologist from St. Louis, and his colleagues published a monograph, *Diseases of the External Ear* as part of the American Lecture Series by Charles C. Thomas Publishers.[1] This work was largely based on numerous research projects on infections of the external auditory canal. They were somewhat motivated by the experience of seeing many soldiers returning from the Pacific in World War II with infections of the external auditory canal. They attempted to elucidate the causes and recommend appropriate antibiotic therapy. Research by various scientists identified mixed flora at the usual cause and the general therapy consisted of a solution consisting of a combination of antibiotics effective against Gram-positive and

Department of Otolaryngology, SUNY-Downstate Medical Center, 450 Clarkson Avenue, Brooklyn, NY 11203, USA
E-mail address: lucente@aol.com

Otolaryngol Clin N Am 56 (2023) xix-xx
https://doi.org/10.1016/j.otc.2023.06.008
0030-6665/23/© 2023 Elsevier Inc. All rights reserved.

Gram-negative bacteria within an acid medium. At this time, the Food and Drug Administration was attempting to discourage the use of combinations of medications in order to focus on single-drug therapy. Senturia testified in Washington and was successful in getting the idea of the combination of antibiotics approved.

I had the pleasure of working with Dr Senturia while serving a resident in Otolaryngology at Washington University in St Louis. It was from the mentorship that I became interested in diseases of the external ear, and, throughout my career, it was a major focus of my practice. In 1980, Dr Senturia, Morris D. Marcus, and I published an extensively expanded text which included much of the original work that was in his 1957 edition and added articles on tumors, trauma, foreign bodies, metabolic diseases, malformations, psychocutaneous diseases, geriatric changes and allergic disorders.[2]

In 1995, I was joined by William Lawson and Nelson Lee Novick in publishing an updated monograph, *The External Ear*,[3] which resulted in an attempt to provide an otologic-dermatologic background for understanding the diverse disorders of the external ear, with more discussion of various surgical procedures that are used in the area.

Treatment of external ear afflictions, long the province of otologists, now involves other professionals including audiologists and other physicians. This has posed a challenge to the otologic community with regard to training of their colleagues and, as time, competitors, as well as in monitoring the results and dealing with any complications.

The recent introduction of over-the-counter hearing aids, self-cleaning devices for removal of cerumen, and self-administered solutions which purport to dissolve wax have taken the professional community into another area of challenges. This is based on the frequent misunderstanding of the role of cerumen.

Cerumen (or ear wax as the public and commercial world frequently refer to it) is an important defense mechanism for the ear. It lubricates the canal and has antibacterial properties which help to prevent infections. It is not dirt! If undisturbed and undeterred, the ear canal skin will generally allow the wax to migrate toward the canal opening where it can be easily removed. However, if the individual used instruments, fingers, cotton swabs or other devices to try to clean the canal, they will generally push the was deeper. These devises can also injure the skin of the canal and even damage the eardrum, if done too vigorously.

Experience has taught that despite one's best efforts, the canal can become completely blocked with wax, producing hearing loss. In these instances, it is prudent for the problem to be handled by an ear care professional who can safely remove the wax, generally under microscopic control, while protecting both the canal skin and tympanic membrane.

The diagnosis and treatment of various conditions involving the external ear canal and auricle continues to evolve. We have generally benefitted from advance in technology, pharmacology, and education. It remains to be seen how the latest challenges will be met. Having studied this area for over 50 years, this author looks forward to following all of the developments.

REFERENCES

1. Senturia BH. Diseases if the external ear. Springfield (IL): Charles C. Thomas Publisher; 1957.
2. Senturia BH, Marcus MD, Lucente FE. Diseases of the external ear: an otologic-dermatologic manual. 2nd edition. New York: Grune and Stratton, Inc.; 1980.
3. Lucente FE, Lawson W, Novick NL. The external ear. New York: WB Saunders Inc; 1995.

The External Auditory Canal
Examination and Evaluation

Matthew B. Hanson, MD

KEYWORDS

- Ear wax • Ear cleaning • Tinnitus

KEY POINTS

- Examination of the external ear can be done with a headlight, a handheld otoscope, an endoscope, or an operating microscope depending on the preference of the examiner.
- For cleaning the ear, a hybrid technique can be used where the substance in the canal can be softened with drops before removal with suction under direct vision.
- The skin of the ear canal should be inspected for pathologic changes.
- Growths in the canal should be inspected and palpated to see if they are soft tissue or bone.

In the world of Otolaryngology–Head and Neck Surgery, the external auditory canal gets scant attention or respect. My mentor, Frank Lucente, MD, has referred to it as the "Rodney Dangerfield of ENT" (in reference to the late comedian who had the ongoing bit of "I don't get no respect..."). On most days, it is nothing more than the tunnel through which we visualize the "real" parts of the ear—the tympanic membrane and the middle ear. Or it is the region that must be cleared of impacted wax or debris from careless overuse of cotton swabs so we can really know how well a patient can hear. The external ear is a real pain.

The external ear is also the focus of many of the complaints for which our patients seek attention from an otolaryngologist. When a patient comes with hearing loss, ear fullness, ear pain, ear itchiness, otorrhea, tinnitus, or any number of other ear complaints, the external canal is often the first place to look for the problem. It is also the one part of the ear that is most easily probed or self-treated by the patient, and thus, the problems found will often have been self-inflicted.

Yet, the external auditory canal is an amazing structure that has evolved to perform a specific function to which it is perfectly suited. It is designed to conduct sound to the eardrum where it is transferred to the inner ear, where it is converted into the nerve impulses, allowing us to perceive the subtle variances in frequency, intensity, harmonics, timbre, and changes in these properties over time to allow humans to decode

Department of Otolaryngology, SUNY, SUNY Downstate College of Medicine, Otolaryngology, Kings County Hospital Center, 450 Clarkson Avenue, PO Box 126, Brooklyn, NY 11203, USA
E-mail address: matthew.hanson@downstate.edu

Otolaryngol Clin N Am 56 (2023) 859–862
https://doi.org/10.1016/j.otc.2023.06.011
0030-6665/23/© 2023 Elsevier Inc. All rights reserved.

meaning from speech and environmental sounds and have a precise concept of where that sound is in relationship to the listener.[1]

A price is paid for this ability. To provide the necessary resonance needed in the all-important human speech frequencies and the directional resonance to allow us to locate a sound along a vertical axis, our ear canal must have an oddly-shaped cartilaginous collecting structure and a long canal with the eardrum and middle ear embedded deep within the temporal bone. As a skin appendage, it will need to be lined by keratinizing squamous epithelium. This epithelial tissue, an ideal protective layer, is in a constant state of regeneration, with new cells being added by the basal layer as the outer cells age, die and detach in a continuous shower of keratin. The ear canal thus requires a process to remove this dead debris, lest it block the canal and prevent our being able to hear. It will also need a way to protect itself from bacteria, fungi, vermin, toxins, and other irritants that would normally be attracted to such a warm and inaccessible environment.

For this reason, the ear canal has evolved an elaborate mechanism that allows this vulnerable area to be protected and continuously cleaned. The layers of the keratinizing epithelium migrate laterally as they mature, creating a continuous river of keratin that migrates away from the eardrum and out of the canal. As this river of keratin reaches the cartilaginous canal, adnexal skin structures, sebaceous glands, apocrine cerumen glands, and hairs that point outward, will lift and emulsify the keratin as it desquamates, degrade it and extrude it out of the ear as a continual flow of ear wax. This mechanism repels water, maintains an acidic environment unfriendly to insects, bacteria, and yeasts, and keeps the ear canal dry and safe, and above all, open and able to permit the transmission of sound. It can easily be supposed that all pathology that affects the ear canal can be traced to a breakdown of this protective mechanism and subsequent restoration of it will address discomfort.

ASSESSMENT OF THE EXTERNAL EAR

As always, we begin patient assessment with the history. For disorders of the ear, there are a limited number of potential patient complaints. Hearing loss, tinnitus, dizziness, and ear drainage are the main ones typically made. Although any of these common symptoms can occur with disease of the external auditory canal, we are more often confronted with less-easily defined sensations, such as ear pain, feeling of fullness or pressure, and the ever-annoying itching and sensation of something crawling in the ear (formication).

When considering the variety of sensations that can be felt in the ears of our patients, the source does not necessarily have to be the ear. Pain, itching, and ear fullness can arise from three broad sources. The first, and most obvious area, is the ear itself. Each of these sensations can arise from disorders of the external, middle, or even the inner ear. Yet, these sensations can also arise as a referred sensation from other areas. Itching is a frequent complaint in patients with seasonal allergic rhinitis, and the use of nasal steroids will often relieve this symptom. A third consideration as a source for ear sensations is those structures close to the ear. The temporomandibular joint is a particularly plentiful source of disturbing ear sensations. Consideration of this paradigm while assessing patient complaints (the ear, a referred sensation, or structure close to the ear) will help to locate the source and reiterates the importance of a complete head and neck evaluation in every patient.

Examination of the external ear can be done with a headlight, a handheld otoscope, an endoscope, or an operating microscope depending on the preference of the examiner. The headlight and the microscope allow both hands to be used for examination and cleaning of the ear. Only the microscope, however, allows the clear visualization of the debris and the tissue that is in the canal. The use of a speculum allows atraumatic straightening of the canal by displacing the cartilaginous canal posteriorly to expose the entire canal. It is important that the speculum be placed after the meatus, or outer opening of the ear canal, is inspected as often dermatologic conditions are most easily identified in this region.

A thorough cleaning of the ear is important in the assessment of the external canal, but before this is begun, the examiner should note the nature and amount of any debris in the canal and note the character of the skin. Often, we call any debris we find in the ear canal "wax," but this is not always so. The soft, brown substance we call "wet wax" or the dry flaky form we call "dry wax" is normal findings in most cases and should only be encountered in the lateral cartilaginous portion of the ear canal. If it is impacted deeply, it has probably been pushed there by the patient trying to clear the ear. Sometimes, what we find deep in the ear is not wax but some other substance. Dried mucus or pus can build up on the wall of the ear canal and look like wax. A large colony of yeast or a plug of desquamated keratin can have a white, creamy appearance or a scaly cast-like appearance. Often it is necessary to remove this debris to see the true pathology. Thus, cleaning of the ear is paramount to diagnosing the problem.

CLEANING THE EAR

In 2008, the American Academy of Otolaryngology Head and Neck Surgery came out with evidence-based practice guidelines for the removal of earwax,[1] and these recommendations were updated in 2017.[2,3] This became one of the most heavily cited articles this publication ever had. In this guideline, the participants reviewed all the evidence and could find no evidence to support the use of one method over another for the removal of earwax. The use of cerumenolytic drops, of which there are many varieties, can significantly soften wax, but the softened wax must then be removed, either by the process of time or active removal in some way. Irrigation, a time-honored technique, can be very effective and comfortable for the patient provided the correct technique is used. Incorrect technique can result in patient pain and injury. It is also a "blind" technique, where the debris removal is not done under direct vision and often the examiner is uncertain of the status of the tympanic membrane. As such, it should be used with caution. Manual removal under direct vision with instruments takes certain skill, and the practitioner must have appropriate visualization and instruments to avoid injury. For the otologic surgeon, however, direct visualization and removal under the microscope using micro instruments is the technique of choice. For the otolaryngologist-in-training, learning to clean out an ear under the microscope without causing discomfort to the patient is a skill that must be mastered for the assessment of diseases of the ear. It is also a skill that will serve the resident in gaining experience with operating using a microscope.

The importance of a clean ear is twofold: it will remove debris that may hide the pathology and it will improve the penetration, and thus the effectiveness, of any drops. All debris needs to be removed—not just cerumen, but dried pus and keratin and any other substance that is not living tissue. Very often, a harmless-appearing piece of wax or crust on the wall of the ear canal may turn out to hide a canal cholesteatoma or other lesion that would otherwise go unnoticed. Trails of dried mucus may lead the way to a perforation or retraction in the tympanic membrane. Many species of yeast secrete a thick glycoprotein biofilm that will make a hard cast that coats the entire medial ear canal and tympanic membrane. Until this is removed, topical treatment will be ineffective.

EXAMINING THE EAR CANAL

Once the ear is cleaned and the tympanic membrane (TM) is seen to be intact, the skin of the ear canal should be inspected for pathologic changes. Erythema and swelling are the hallmarks of an acute otitis externa. Hyper keratosis and thickening, particularly at the lateral meatus of the ear canal, suggest a dermatitis. Growths in the canal should be inspected and palpated to see if they are soft tissue or bone.

In most cases of disease of the external ear, cleaning and inspection are enough to direct empirical therapy or further workup. Biopsy, culture, and radiology will be helpful in many situations.

CLINICS CARE POINTS

- All physical assessment in patients with ear complaints must begin with a thorough cleaning and examination of the exteranl auditory canal.
- there are many techniques and variations in how to examine and clean the ear canal. Evidence does not support any ne . Choice of technique is determined by the skill of the examiner, the nature of the problem and the least discomfort for the patient.

DISCLOSURE

The author has no conflicts of interest.

REFERENCES

1. Balachanda BB. Theoretical and applied external ear acoustics. J Am Acad Audiol 1997;8(6):411–20.
2. Roland P, Smith T, Schwartz S, et al. Clinical practice guideline: cerumen impaction. Otolaryngol Head Neck Surg 2008;139(3 suppl 2):S1–21.
3. Schwartz S, Magit AE, Rosenfeld RM, et al. Clinical practice guideline (update): Earwax (cerumen impaction). Otolaryngol Head Neck Surg 2017;156(Suppl 1): S1–29.

Follow the Wax
The Natural Protection of the Ear Canal and Its Biome

Matthew B. Hanson, MD[a],*, Matthew Adams, MD[b]

KEYWORDS

- Ear canal • Wet wax • External auditory canal

KEY POINTS

- The external auditory canal is a complex structure that is perfectly suited for its function.
- The skin of the deep bony ear canal has a migratory function that moves laterally in the ear canal over time.
- The properties of earwax and the normal ear canal biome help protect the ear from pathologic conditions.

CANAL SKIN MIGRATION

It had been long known that the ear canal skin has a migratory characteristic. Initial studies of this were carried out as far back as 1882[1] and were dramatically demonstrated by the "ink dot" experiments of Alberti in 1964,[2] where the rate of epithelial migration averaged 0.05 mm/d, but it varied depending on the quadrant studied. The external ear canal is a skin appendage and, like the rest of our skin, is covered by keratinizing squamous epithelium. The principal characteristic of this epithelium is the continuous creation of a water-tight layer of desquamating squamous cells (the epidermis) created by an underlying and stable basal cell layer (the dermis). Only the basal and granular cells of the epidermis are capable of division, and all other layers (stratum spinosum, stratum lucidum, and stratum corneum) represent stages of conversion to the thin, desquamating corneal layer. On the outside of the body, the outermost layers of skin flake off onto our clothes and into the air. But the ear canal is a blind cul-de-sac at the end of which is the tympanic membrane. The function of the tympanic membrane depends on its mobility, which would be compromised by

[a] Department of Otolaryngology, SUNY, SUNY Downstate College of Medicine, Kings County Hospital Center, 450 Clarkson Avenue, PO Box 126, Brooklyn, NY 11203, USA; [b] Resident Physician, Departmentof Otolaryngology, SUNY Downstate Medical Center, 450 Clarkson Avenue, Box 126, Brooklyn, NY 11203, USA
* Corresponding author.
E-mail address: matthew.hanson@downstate.edu

Otolaryngol Clin N Am 56 (2023) 863–867
https://doi.org/10.1016/j.otc.2023.06.005
0030-6665/23/© 2023 Elsevier Inc. All rights reserved.

a thick layer of epidermis, and the ear canal would be fully occluded by desquamated skin in about 3 months if it were not for the process of this continuous migration.

The exact mechanism of the migration is not fully known and likely has to do with a directional division of the cells that will direct the daughter cell in a direction away from the epicenter of the migration, the umbo of the malleus. The basal cells also migrate but much slower than the stratum corneum. There is also evidence for an active directional growth pattern of the entire epidermis, like that seen in the production of the fingernails, and the desquamated cells tend to be elongated in the direction of migration, implying a role of the cytoskeleton in migration.[3]

The migratory character of the canal epithelium is characteristic only of the skin of the medial, bony canal. The skin of the bony canal is thin and attaches directly to the periosteum of the bone with no papillae and no adnexal tissue. As the migration reaches the cartilaginous canal, the subcutaneous tissue becomes more plentiful, and there are hairs and glandular structures. The hairs of the cartilaginous canal are pointed outward and act as a "ramp" to elevate the desquamated keratin. The glands are of two types, sebaceous glands, which are usually subcutaneous and associated with hairs, and apocrine "cerumen" glands. There are no eccrine sweat glands in the external canal. Sebaceous secretion is a fatty substance that is passively secreted into the base of the hair cells and help to emulsify the keratin and facilitate its continued migration. Apocrine secretions are whole-cell secretions that have a milky character. These three substances, the desquamated keratin, sebum, and apocrine secretions, make up the bulk of what we term "ear wax."

Components and Properties of Ear Wax

The bulk of the mass of ear wax is made from desquamated keratin, sebum secreted from sebaceous glands, and the secretion from the apocrine cerumen glands. The keratin is a water-resistant nonliving and tightly connected substance that is what is left of the skin of the deep ear canal. The sebaceous secretions are the typical high-lipid content secretions that are characteristic of this gland elsewhere in the body.

The apocrine glands, on the other hand, are a unique structure of the external ear and have a variety of properties of its secretions. These glands are coiled tubes with their secretions being directly drained into the hair follicle.[4] The glandular cells are tall and elongated, and their apical protrusions are pinched off into the lumen of the duct for secretion. There are numerous mast cells and IgA-positive plasma cells associated with the cerumen glands, and the secretions are positive for IgA. There is also secretion of several proteins with antimicrobial properties, including lactoferrin, lysozyme, mucin, cathelicidin, and beta-defensin. It is the differences in the structure of the ceruminous glands that differentiate wet wax from dry wax.[5]

The issue of wet wax versus dry wax has been an issue of much scientific investigation over the past several years. There is a strong ethnic variance in the frequency of each with wet wax predominant in African and Caucasian races and dry wax predominating in Asian populations. Linkage studies have found this to be a single-gene trait, with the gene located in the pericentromeric region of chromosome 16.[6] In 2006, Yoshiura and colleagues traced the difference to a single-nucleotide polymorphism in the gene for ABCC11 (ATP-binding cassette transporter sub-family C, member 11) also known as MRP8 (multidrug resistance related protein-8).[7] The substitution of an adenine nucleotide at the 538 position (538G- > A) will result in dry earwax in a homozygote. Persons with heterozygote AG or homozygote GG will have wet wax. This was the first instance ever where a single-nucleotide polymorphism was found to result in an easily-identifiable trait. The product of this class of genes is known to be a lipophilic anion pump. This genetic determinant has also been implicated in risk of breast cancer[8] and in axillary odor[9] as the glands of the breast and the sweat glands of the axillae are also modified apocrine glands.

The components of earwax make it an important part of the protective immunity of the ear canal. The lipophilic nature repels water and helps keep the ear canal dry. The low pH of wax suppresses the growth of bacterial species and is unpleasant to insects. The antibiotic properties can further prevent infections. In summary, earwax is good stuff.

The Biome of the External Canal

One aspect of the external ear and of earwax that is often forgotten about, however, is the enormous number of species that call our ear canals home. The external auditory canal is a highly specialized appendage of the integumental system of the exterior of our body. As such, it is home to an enormous variety of organisms of multiple different types. Most of the time, the organisms are commensal (ie, live together with no harm done to either species), but many times, it is symbiotic (where the relationship of organism and host is mutually beneficial) and only rarely is it pathologic.

Initial studies of the external ear microbiome were performed using standard microbiologic culturing techniques.[10] These showed a wide variety of bacterial species cultured from normal ears, including Staphylococcus epidermidis, Corynebacterium, Staphylococcus aureus, Escherichia coli, and Streptococcus pyogenes. Pseudomonas species were rarely cultured, and fungi were rare in these cultured specimens. The use of culture techniques, however, will often underestimate the population of fastidious organisms (organisms difficult to culture) and organisms the reside in specific adnexal structures.

Next-generation DNA sequencing has dramatically changed our understanding of the normal human biome.[11] This uses PCR-amplification of DNA to identify and sequence the 16S ribosomal RNA to allow a very accurate and quantitative assessment of all microbiologic populations, no matter how fastidious. Studies using this technique in the external ear showed a wide variety of organisms, even those not identified in previous culture-based studies.[12] It also shows a marked decrease in the biodiversity during acute infection with Staphylococcus, Corynebacterium, and Pseudomonas species accounting for most species.

The bacterial microbiome of the external ear is only part of the story, and similar microbiologic techniques are being used to identify the populations of fungi and animal residents as well. PCR amplification of the D1/D2 regions of the rRNA large subunit has shown an ample population of fungi in a normal ear canal. Most of these are of the species of Malassezia, a very fastidious and lipid-requiring variety of yeast.[13] Malassezia is a genus of yeast that cannot make certain lipids, and as such, their survival requires they have a constant source of lipids. The species of Malassezia are ubiquitous in the sebaceous glands of all species and are considered a commensal and symbiotic organism. However, Malassezia has also been implicated in several dermatologic conditions, most notably pityriasis versicolor and seborrheic dermatitis.[14] What turns this normally commensal organism into a pathogen is unknown but is believed to be an increased immune-reactivity to the species.

In addition to fungi, there are also other microorganisms that inhabit the external canal. Demodex mite is an obligate human ecto-parasite that resides in the pilosebaceous units of our skin and, in most cases, causes no symptoms.[15] It has, however, been implicated in cases of ear pruritus and will often worsen if steroids are used.[16]

SUMMARY

The external auditory canal is a complex structure that is perfectly suited for its function. The skin of the deep bony ear canal has a migratory function that moves laterally in the ear canal over time. As it reaches the cartilaginous ear canal, the keratin of the ear canal is lifted up by the hairs and is emulsified by the secretions of the sebaceous and apocrine cerumen glands to create earwax. The properties of that earwax and the normal ear canal biome help protect the ear from pathologic conditions, and it is often the overremoval of this protective element that increases the risk of external ear infections.

CLINICS CARE POINTS

- Ear wax is a complex substance that functions to protect and clean the external ear canal.
- Ear wax has properties that suppress the growth of harmful microbes while maintaining the beneficial microbes of its biome.

DISCLOSURE

The authors have no conflicts of interest.

REFERENCES

1. Blake CJ. Progressive growth of the dermoid coat of the tympanic membrane. Am J Otol 1882;266–8.
2. Alberti PWR. Epithelial migration of the tympanic membrane. J Laryngol Otol 1964;78:808–30.
3. Johnson A, Hawke M. Cell shape in the migratory epidermis of the external auditory canal. J Otolaryngol 1985;14:273–81.
4. Stoeckelhuber M, Matthias C, Andratschke M, et al. Human ceruminous gland: Ultrastructureall and histochemical analysis of antimicrobial and cytoskeletal components. Anat Rec 2006;288A:877–84.
5. Shugyo Y, Sudo N, Kanai Y, et al. Morphological differences between secretory cells of wet and dry types of human ceruminous glands. Am J Anat 1988;181: 377–84.
6. Tomita H, Yamada K, Ghadami M, et al. Mapping of the wet/dry earwax locus to the pericentromeric region of chromosome 16. Lancet 2002;359(9322): 2000–2.
7. Yoshiura K, Kinoshita A, Ishida T, et al. A SNP in the ABCC11 gene is the determinant of human earwax type. Nat Genet 2006;38(3):324–30.
8. Petrakis NL, King EB, Lee M, et al. Cerumen phenotype and preliferative epithelium in breast fluid of U.S.-born vs. immigrant Asian women:a possible genetic-environmental interaction. Breast Cance Res Treat 1990;16(3): 279–85.
9. Nakano M, Miwa N, Hirano A, et al. A strong association of axillary osmidrosis with wet earwax type determined by genotyping of the ABCC11 gene. BMC Genet 2009;10:42.
10. Perry ET, Nichols AC. Studies on the growth of bacteria in the human ear canal. J Invest Dermatol 1956;27:165.

11. Turnbaugh PJ, Ley RE, Hamady M, et al. The human microbiome project. Nature 2007;449:804–10.
12. Kim S, Han SJ, Hong SJ, et al, Microbiome of acute otitis externa. J Clin Med 2022;11:7074.
13. Cho O, Sugita T. Comprehensive Analysis of the fungal microbiota of the human external auditory canal using pyrosequencing: The external auditory canal exhibits low fungal species diversity. Med Mycol J 2017; 58E:E1–4.
14. Ashbee HR. Update on the genus Malassezia. Med Mycol 2007;45:287–303.
15. Rather P, Hassan I. Human Demodex Mite: *The versatile mite of dermatologic importance.* Indian J Dermatol 2014;59(1):60–6.
16. Cevik C, Aycan Kay O, Akbay E, et al. Investigation of demodex species frequency in patients with persisten itchy ears canal treated with local steroid. J Laryngol Otol 2014;128(8):698–701.

"Do-It-Yourself" Ear Canal Care

Donald Tan, MD[a], Jacob B. Hunter, MD[b],*

KEYWORDS

- Ear cleaning • Home ear care • Ear cleaning products • Ear cleaning devices
- Ear wax • Cerumen • Cerumen impaction • Home cerumen remedy

KEY POINTS

- There is limited evidence to support the safety or efficacy of all types of "do-it-yourself" home cerumen removal methods.
- The American Academy of Otolaryngology–Head and Neck Surgery recommends patients do not place any objects in their ears, and that select patients can consider trying alcohol or hydrogen peroxide drops/irrigation, topical ear wax softening agents, or irrigation with bulb syringe or irrigation kits.
- There are no premarket regulatory mechanisms in place for commercially available ear cleaning products, although consumers may independently report adverse outcomes to the Food and Drug Administration or Consumer Product Safety Commission.

 Video content accompanies this article at http://www.oto.theclinics.com.

INTRODUCTION

The current marketplace of commercially available "do-it-yourself" at-home ear cleaning devices ranges from benign to bizarre to downright hazardous. With a single exception (ear candles), these devices are considered a "convenience kit" by the Food and Drug Administration (FDA) and therefore are exempt from premarket notification, not requiring a demonstration of safety or efficacy to be sold in the United States. Consumers who are injured by the devices theoretically have the option of independently filing a complaint with the FDA or the Consumer Product Safety Commission (CPSC); however, these data are not tracked by any entity and are difficult to access by consumers. As a result, most otolaryngologists are routinely asked by their patients to comment on the safety and efficacy of devices that many practitioners

[a] Department of Otolaryngology–Head and Neck Surgery, University of Texas Southwestern Medical Center, 2001 Inwood Road, Dallas, TX 75390, USA; [b] Department of Otolaryngology–Head and Neck Surgery, Thomas Jefferson University Hospital, 925 Chestnut Street, Philadelphia, PA 19017, USA
* Corresponding author.
E-mail address: Jacob.Hunter@jefferson.edu

Otolaryngol Clin N Am 56 (2023) 869–879
https://doi.org/10.1016/j.otc.2023.06.009
0030-6665/23/© 2023 Elsevier Inc. All rights reserved.
oto.theclinics.com

have never heard of and for which safety/efficacy data likely do not exist. In this article, the authors aim to provide a broad overview of the types of devices available on the market and some general considerations regarding their usage.

DISCUSSION
Blind Instruments

The American Academy of Otolaryngology–Head and Neck Surgery (AAO-HNS) Clinical Practice Guideline (CPG) on Cerumen Impaction recommends clinicians advise patients to avoid placing anything in their ear that is smaller than their elbow.[1] Blind instrumentation may lead to canal laceration, secondary infection, tympanic membrane perforation, ossicular chain disruption, hearing loss, vertigo, bleeding, and so forth. However, there are scant objective data available on the rates of self-induced injury related to blind instrumentation of the ear. In a survey of 141 Nigerian health care workers, 129 subjects admitted to ear cleaning by various methods, 12 (9.3%) of which reported associated ear injuries.[2] Despite the theoretical danger, there are a wide variety of commercially available products intended for manual cerumen removal without visual guidance. A general knowledge of the available products can help counsel patients who cannot be dissuaded from manually cleaning their ears routinely.

Cotton-tipped applicator (CTA) usage for self-ear hygiene has become equal parts epidemic and cultural phenomenon. The well-recognized "Q-tips" were first introduced to the market by Leo Gerstenzang in 1923 for the purpose of various hygiene tasks for infants. Sometime in the 1970s their labeling began to include warnings against inserting into the ear canal.[3] Between 1990 and 2010, an estimated 263,338 children aged less than 18 years were treated for CTA-related ear injuries in US hospital emergency departments.[4] Nearly every commercially available ear cleaning device markets themselves as a safer and more effective alternative to CTA. Despite the manufacturer, medical professionals, and even commercial competitors warning against the usage of CTA in the ear canal, the practice remains widespread because of cultural and/or familial beliefs regarding ear hygiene.

The Ototek Loop (**Fig. 1**) is a plastic cerumen loop with a fixed guard to prevent penetrating tympanic membrane injury.[5] Of note, the design was patented by a Comprehensive Otolaryngologist, Dr Estrem. The plastic material may be safer than metal alternatives in terms of risk of abrading or lacerating the ear canal. It is unclear how effective the guard is given natural variation in the length of the external auditory

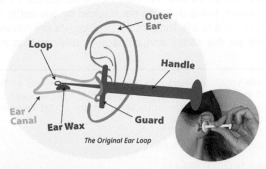

Fig. 1. Instructional schematic from product web site. (Ototek Loop. With permission from Dr. Scott Estrem, MD (Developer).)

canal (EAC); however, the product is intended for use in patients 16 years or older presumably for this reason. Of note, the inventor Dr. Estrem reports over 3 million units sold and no reported instances of significant ear injuries. Similar products exist with different curette material, as well as adjustable guard lengths. As with any blind technique, there is risk for further impaction of cerumen with this device.

The Tvidler Spiral Ear Cleaner (**Fig. 2**) is a silicone tapered spiral-shaped device that is fluted like a drill head.[6] Per the disclaimer Web page, the intended use is for removing excess cerumen from the lateral portion of the EAC in adults only and is not an FDA-approved medical device for the treatment or diagnosis of disease related to cerumen. Assuming patients have no reasonable way of determining the depth of insertion within their own EAC, this device is likely to contribute to further impaction of medial cerumen. This device is unlikely to be helpful for home maintenance in patients with cerumen impaction.

There are a wide variety of metal curette ear cleaning sets available on the market (**Fig. 3**).[7] The sets commonly contain a variety of picks/curettes with different head shapes and lengths. Although CTA usage is a common practice in the West, in some other cultures the metal ear cleaning set is a ubiquitous household item. In Chengdu, China, professional ear cleaners roam in public spaces and offer ear cleaning with a variety of picks as a commercial service.[8] Despite how widespread this practice is globally, there is insufficient evidence to conclude whether the practice of ear cleaning under direct visualization by another is a safe or effective treatment for cerumen impaction.

DROPS

The CPG concludes that although empirical evidence to support instilling prophylactic topical solutions for the prevention of cerumen impaction is limited, it is an option to discuss with patients.[1] Many "cerumenolytic" agents are described in the literature that may be broadly categorized as water-based, oil-based, or other (nonwater, non-oil-based). Oil-based preparations aim to loosen wax by dissolving it in oil. Water-based and other preparations aim to increase the wax's ability to dissolve in water (miscibility).[9] A single study comparing olive oil spray to no treatment found olive oil increased the weight of ear canal contents compared with the untreated ear.[10] Therefore, olive oil is the only topical solution not advised by the AAO-HNS. A 2018 Cochrane Review comparing the efficacy of cerumenolytic agents concluded that

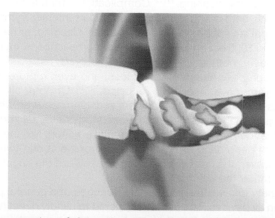

Fig. 2. Digital representation of theoretical device function from product web site. (*From* tvidler.com.)

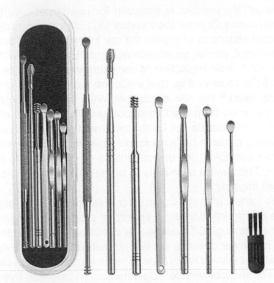

Fig. 3. Metal ear curette kit. (*From* Amazon.com.)

(1) no high-quality evidence showed one agent is more effective than another; (2) only a single study concluded that treatment with drops is more effective than no treatment; (3) there was insufficient evidence to compare water/saline with cerumenolytics or no treatment; (4) adverse events were rare and mild.[9] In addition, there is little evidence to suggest an ideal frequency or duration of the above treatments. In summary, topical solutions pose minimal risk to patients with intact tympanic membranes and provide the possibility of benefit for treating cerumen impaction.

IRRIGATION SYSTEMS

Ear syringing with the intention of displacing earwax via hydraulic pressure is commonplace, and a variety of products are commercially available. These range from syringes requiring manual generation of pressure (**Figs. 4** and **5**) to powered irrigators intended for dental cleaning.[11,12] Complications, both minor and severe, have been described with both manual and powered instruments. Tympanic membrane perforation, ear canal laceration, infection of the ear, bleeding, or hearing loss occurs at a rate of about 1 in 1000 ear irrigations.[1] Serious complications, including immediate temporary and delayed permanent facial nerve paralysis, ossicular chain disruption, perilymph fistula, complete audiovestibular loss, and even rupture of an internal carotid artery aneurysm, have also been reported.[13–16] Of note, all of the previously mentioned serious complications related to ear syringing occurred with a provider performing the syringing on the patient. A cadaveric study of dental irrigators conducted in 1991 showed that commercially available dental irrigators like the Teledyne Waterpik were capable of perforating the tympanic membrane at one-third of the maximal power setting; however, the risk of perforation was lower if the irrigator tip was angled toward the canal rather than straight.[15]

Despite the variety in over-the-counter ear syringes, the general principle remains the same between all devices. The user is expected to blindly direct a manually generated column of water pressure into their ear without occluding the canal with the syringe so that there is a pathway for egress of effluent. Accidental occlusion of the canal

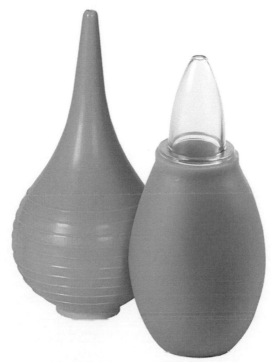

Fig. 4. Manual bulb syringe for ear irrigation. (Ezy Dose Kids® Ear Syringe & Nasal Aspirator. With permission from Apothecary Products, LLC.)

with the device during usage can generate significant pressure on the tympanic membrane, which has been associated with serious injury, as mentioned previously. The available manual devices tend to be more affordable than powered options.

WUSH

The Wush ear cleaner (**Fig. 6**) is a battery-powered device, which features 3 water streams that aim toward the ear canal and a variety of power settings for irrigation.[17] The cleaner claims to be a safe and doctor-recommended alternative to the ineffective CTA, but like all other ear cleaning devices, it is exempt from premarket notification with the FDA. Although there are no one-star reviews on the product Web site, a review of 98 one-star reviews on Amazon.com reveals minor complications that are common to all irrigation methods, that is, vertigo, tinnitus, acquired otitis externa, failure to resolve impaction, but at the time of this writing, there was no mention of traumatic tympanic membrane perforations or other serious complications.[18]

OtoSet

The OtoSet (SafKan Health, USA) (**Fig. 7**) is not available for over-the-counter purchase and is intended for use by health care professionals in a clinical setting only, but is worth mentioning as a potential future "do-it-yourself" option.[19] Per the manufacturer, "OtoSet is the first automated and FDA-cleared ear cleaning device for clinical use. In a 30-second cleaning cycle, irrigation is directed from solution containers through disposable ear tips and towards the walls of the ear canals to break down earwax. Continuous micro-suction draws the earwax and water back through the ear tips and into disposable waste containers for a mess-free procedure."

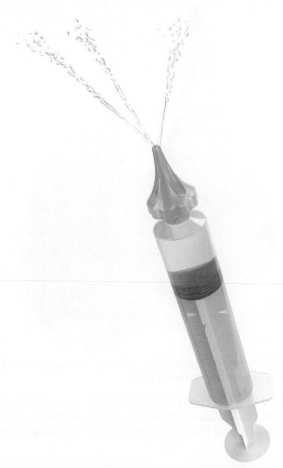

Fig. 5. Manual ear syringe with effluent bucket for ear irrigation. (Earwax Removal Syringe. With permission from Apothecary Products, LLC.)

The FDA approved the device for use by clinicians because the inventors demonstrated "substantial equivalence" to an existing device's safety and effectiveness. Although for context, as CEO Sahil Diwan did state, "Our substantial equivalence was literally a syringe."[20] As the device features simultaneous ingress and egress, it is hoped it will be safer than manual irrigation, which risks accidental formation of seal and resultant tympanic membrane, and potentially middle ear, injury.

Video-Assisted Instruments

A recent trend has been the development of over-the-counter endoscopes with ear cleaning attachments fitted to the end of the camera with the ability to transmit video to phones/tablets. These devices also fall under the category of "items smaller than your elbow" and are not recommended for use by the AAO-HNS. Theoretically, the ability to provide direct visualization to the user should improve safety when compared with blind instrumentation. However, learning to perform procedures in a 3-dimensional space using a 2-dimensional image is a major challenge. In one video review, an Otolaryngologist tried 2 brands of ear cleaning cameras and ultimately deemed

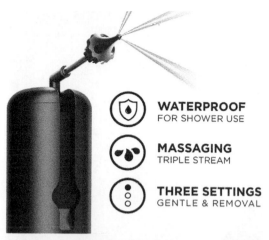

Fig. 6. Wush ear cleaner product description from product web site. (*From* blackwolfnation. com.)

them unsafe and not likely to be effective (Video 1).[21] The cleaning instrument significantly impairs visualization, as pictured in **Fig. 8**.[22] The devices are also significantly wider than standard endoscopic ear instruments, limiting maneuverability within the ear canal as the proximal end of the instrument contacts the ear canal before the instrumented tip. Using the device solely as a camera may have utility for patients in the era of telemedicine.

CANDLING

Ear candling/coning is a cerumen removal method that involves placing a hollow cone-shaped candle into the EAC, igniting it, and removing it just before the flame

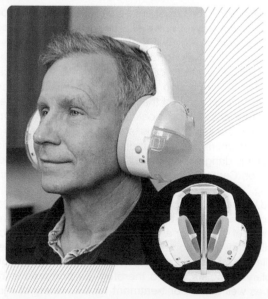

Fig. 7. Otoset ear cleaner in use. (OtoSet®. With permission from SafKan, Inc.)

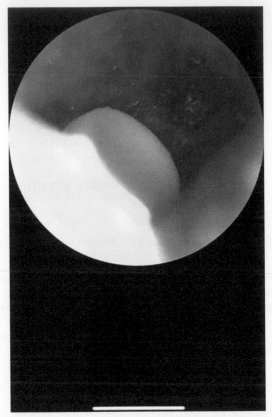

Fig. 8. User-uploaded photograph in review from product web site. (*From* axelglade.com.)

reaches the auricle (**Fig. 9**).[23] The target ear canal contents are purportedly adhered to the tip of the candle at the time of removal. The commonly described mechanism is called "the chimney effect," in which the column of hot air creates a vacuum effect within the EAC. This however has not been demonstrated in tympanometric studies of ear candling.[24] This same study compared the effect of ear candling in 4 ears with and without cerumen impaction and showed no effect on cerumen impaction and candle wax deposition in some of the normal ears. Injuries related to ear candling reported in the literature include "ear blockage, ear canal burns, tympanic membrane perforation, conductive hearing loss, otitis externa, and hair fire."[1] In 2010, the FDA issued a warning to consumers that ear candling has no scientific evidence to support its efficacy and that it is dangerous when used according to its labeling.[25] The AAO-HNS updated CPG on Cerumen Impaction recommends that clinicians recommend against ear candling.[1]

Clinicians should be aware that ear candles remain widely commercially available in the United States despite the FDA requirement that packaging may not contain labeling that they are medical devices or are intended for the purpose of cerumen removal. Practitioners of "alternative" or homeopathic medicine promote the effectiveness of ear candling in relieving common complaints like sinus pressure, otalgia, headache, and allergies. Otolaryngologists should therefore be prepared to dissuade patients from ear candling as well as render treatment for the variety of injuries the practice may cause.

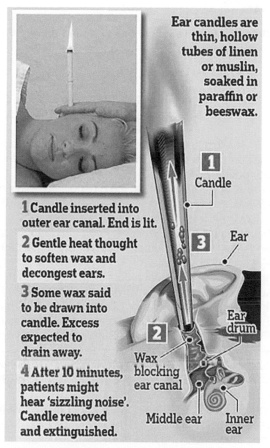

Ear candles are thin, hollow tubes of linen or muslin, soaked in paraffin or beeswax.

1️⃣ Candle

1 Candle inserted into outer ear canal. End is lit.

2 Gentle heat thought to soften wax and decongest ears.

3 Some wax said to be drawn into candle. Excess expected to drain away.

3️⃣ Ear

Ear drum

4 After 10 minutes, patients might hear 'sizzling noise'. Candle removed and extinguished.

2️⃣

Wax blocking ear canal

Middle ear   Inner ear

Fig. 9. Explanation of ear candling from chiropractor's web site. (*From* drcurleychiro.com.)

CLINICS CARE POINTS

- There is limited evidence to support the safety or efficacy of all types of "do-it-yourself" home cerumen removal methods.

- The American Academy of Otolaryngology–Head and Neck Surgery recommends patients do not place any objects in their ears, and that select patients can consider trying alcohol or hydrogen peroxide drops/irrigation, topical ear wax softening agents, or irrigation with bulb syringe or irrigation kits.

- There are no premarket regulatory mechanisms in place for commercially available ear cleaning products, although consumers may independently report adverse outcomes to the Food and Drug Administration or Consumer Product Safety Commission.

DISCLOSURE

The authors declare that they have no relevant or material financial interests that relate to the research described in this article.

SUPPLEMENTARY DATA

Supplementary data related to this article can be found online at https://doi.org/10.1016/j.otc.2023.06.009..

REFERENCES

1. Schwartz SR, Magit AE, Rosenfeld RM, et al. Clinical practice guideline (update): earwax (cerumen impaction). Otolaryngol Head Neck Surg 2017;156(1_suppl): S1–29.
2. Adeyi AA, Tonga LN. What health professionals at the Jos University Teaching Hospital insert in their ears. Niger J Med 2013;22(2):109–12. Available at: http://www.ncbi.nlm.nih.gov/pubmed/23829120.
3. Ferdman RA. The strange life of Q-tips, the most bizarre thing people buy. Available at: https://www.washingtonpost.com/news/wonk/wp/2016/01/20/we-have-a-q-tips-problem/%0A. Accessed March 11, 2023.
4. Ameen ZS, Chounthirath T, Smith GA, et al. Pediatric Cotton-tip applicator-related ear injury treated in united states emergency departments, 1990-2010. J Pediatr 2017;186:124–30.
5. Ototek. Available at: https://ototekloop.com/. Accessed March 11, 2023.
6. Tvidler. Available at: https://tvidler.com/. Accessed March 11, 2023.
7. 8 Pcs Ear Pick Earwax Removal Kit, Ear Cleansing Tool Set, Ear Curette Ear Wax Remover Tool with Cleaning Brush and Storage Box. Available at: https://www.amazon.com/Removal-Cleansing-Curette-Remover-Cleaning/dp/B07Q51DWF6. Accessed March 11, 2023.
8. Hoy H. In China, Chengdu's peculiar ear-cleaning custom. Published 2018. Available at: https://www.bbc.com/travel/article/20181029-in-china-chengdus-peculiar-ear-cleaning-custom. Accessed March 11, 2023.
9. Aaron K, Cooper TE, Warner L, et al. Ear drops for the removal of ear wax. Cochrane Database Syst Rev 2018;7(7):CD012171.
10. Rodgers R. Does olive oil prevent earwax build-up? An experimental study. Pract Nurs 2013;24(4):191–6.
11. Acu-Life Ear and Ear Wax Cleaner for Humans Includes Syringe with Tri-Stream Tip and Ear Wax catching Basin.\ https://www.amazon.com/Cleaner-Humans-Syringe-Tri-Stream-catching/dp/B08VFWTXNN/ref=sr_1_1_sspa?crid=2PA-WHYCLMF30X&keywords=ear+syringe&qid=1677529718&s=hpc&sprefix='''ear+syringe%2Chpc%2C104&sr=1-1-spons&psc=1&spLa=ZW5jcnlwdGV-kUXVhbGlmaWVyPUEyMTYxMjM4SEE5Q0. Accessed March 11, 2023.
12. DMI Baby Nasal Aspirator, Ear Syringe, Mucus Sucker and Nasal Bulb Syringe, 2 Ounces, Blue, 1 Count (Pack of 1), (650-4004-0121). Available at: https://www.amazon.com/Briggs-Nasal-Aspirator-Syringe-Ounce/dp/B001OTK6JG/ref=sr_1_7?crid=2PAWHYCLMF30X&keywords=ear+syringe&qid=1677529718&s=hpc&sprefix=ear+syringe%2Chpc%2C104&sr=1-7. Accessed March 11, 2023.
13. Tshifularo M, Masotja MSL. Ruptured internal carotid artery aneurysm presenting with bloody otorrhoea and epistaxis as a result of ear syringing. S Afr J Surg 2008;46(4):136. Available at: http://www.ncbi.nlm.nih.gov/pubmed/19051956.
14. Ahmed MN, Shetty P, Saunders N, et al. Permanent facial paralysis and hearing loss after aural irrigation. JAMA Otolaryngol Head Neck Surg 2020;146(2):206–8.
15. Dinsdale RC, Roland PS, Manning SC, et al. Catastrophic otologic injury from oral jet irrigation of the external auditory canal. Laryngoscope 1991;101(1 Pt 1):75–8.
16. Thomas AM, Poojary B, Badaridatta HC. Facial nerve palsy as a complication of ear syringing. J Laryngol Otol 2012;126(7):714–6.

17. BlackWolfNation. Available at: https://blackwolfnation.com/pages/specialoffer-fb-v19. Accessed March 11, 2023.
18. Wush Pro by Black Wolf Amazon Reviews. Available at: https://www.amazon.com/Wush-Pro-Black-Wolf-Rechargeable/product-reviews/B09X27SLDB/ref=cm_cr_unknown?ie=UTF8&reviewerType=all_reviews&filterByStar=one_star&pageNumber=1. Accessed March 11, 2023.
19. OtoSet. Available at: https://otoset.com/. Accessed March 11, 2023.
20. Schubert C. Earwax-removal device heads to market with $8M, FDA clearance and a viral TikTok video. Available at: https://www.geekwire.com/2023/earwax-removal-device-heads-to-market-with-8m-fda-clearance-and-a-viral-tiktok-video. Accessed March 11, 2023.
21. Veer V. Ear Surgeon Reviews Home Ear Wax Removal Cameras. Available at: https://www.youtube.com/watch?v=sKuE5Ljrm7A. Accessed March 11, 2023.
22. AxelGlade. Available at: https://www.axelglade.com/products/spade. Accessed March 11, 2023.
23. drcurleychiro. Available at: https://www.drcurleychiro.com/ear-candling-. Accessed March 11, 2023.
24. Seely DR, Quigley SM, Langman AW. Ear candles–efficacy and safety. Laryngoscope 1996;106(10):1226–9.
25. Import Alert 77-01. Available at: https://www.accessdata.fda.gov/cms_ia/importalert_225.html. Accessed March 11, 2023.

Management of Foreign Bodies in the Ear Canal

Steven D. Curry, MD, Anne K. Maxwell, MD*

KEYWORDS

- Foreign body • Ear • Ear canal • External auditory canal • Button batteries
- Otology

KEY POINTS

- Forceps are useful for graspable objects and are often used by emergency physicians without referral to an otolaryngologist.
- Binocular microscopy with microinstrumentation, including angled hooks and currettes, is useful for hard, spherical objects, though general anesthesia may be required in an uncooperative patient.
- Remove button batteries urgently; otic drops and irrigation are strictly contraindicated.
- Douse live insects preferentially in mineral oil prior to removal, as lidocaine in the presence of a TM perforation can cause severe vertigo.

INTRODUCTION

Aural foreign bodies can be found in all ages, with the highest number in preschool-aged children. Suspicion for aural foreign body may arise due to witnessed insertion, visible foreign body, otalgia, aural fullness, muffled hearing, pruritis, bleeding, tinnitus, or, less commonly, chronic cough due to stimulation of Arnold's branch of the vagal nerve.[1,2] In one large study of 17,325 aural foreign bodies, 85.6% were found in children, most commonly aged 1 to 4 years, while 14.1% were removed from adults.[3] While the most common aural foreign bodies vary across geographic locations, jewelry (especially earrings), paper, seeds, stones, insects, plastic toys and beads, and cotton buds are most common in children, with cotton buds most commonly found in adult ears.[1,4] As children age, plastic toys and stones decrease in frequency, while cotton buds and insects increase.[5]

Instrumentation to best remove an aural foreign body varies with its size, location, shape, and consistency. The sigmoidal shape of the external auditory canal (EAC) can make removal challenging, with natural stenoses at the bony-cartilaginous

Department of Otolaryngology-Head and Neck Surgery, University of Nebraska Medical Center, 981225 Nebraska Medical Center, Omaha, NE 68198-1225, USA
* Corresponding author.
E-mail address: anmaxwell@unmc.edu

Otolaryngol Clin N Am 56 (2023) 881–889
https://doi.org/10.1016/j.otc.2023.06.002

junction and lateral to the annulus. Emergency department (ED) physicians can often remove aural foreign bodies, but studies report increased rates of complications with removal by a nonotolaryngologist and decreased tolerance of subsequent attempts, increasing the need for general anesthesia.[5,6] If not readily removable by an ED or primary care physician, referral to an otolaryngologist has been recommended.[6]

EVALUATION

Evaluation should consist of a comprehensive history and head and neck physical examination paying special attention to both ears and nasal cavities. Tuning fork testing can be helpful if the patient is able to participate. It is not uncommon for children to present with more than one foreign body. Therefore, both the ears and the nasal cavities should be examined. Notably, nasal foreign body presentation may be delayed, such that malodorous nasal discharge, especially when unilateral, should be treated as a foreign body until proven otherwise. Nasal foreign bodies should be removed expeditiously to avoid migration/aspiration and airway obstruction.

MANAGEMENT
Instruments, Techniques, and Challenges of EAC Foreign Body Removal

As with other otologic procedures, the best outcomes in the removal of EAC foreign bodies occur with using the correct instruments, binocular microscopy, and a cooperative, restrained, or, if necessary, sedated patient. Instruments have advantages and disadvantages based on the type of foreign body, its shape, size, and position in the EAC.[7,8] **Table 1** summarizes commonly used instruments. Beyond removal of the foreign body itself, the goals should be to avoid repeated attempts, reduce trauma or complication, and avoid introducing an additional, iatrogenic foreign body in the process.

Foreign bodies with a graspable surface or edge, such as paper, cloth, hearing aid domes, earrings, and cotton, can be grasped with alligator or Hartman foreign body forceps and removed.[9] Alligator forceps are ideal for grasping thin edges, while Hartman forceps are able to accommodate larger items.

Spherical and/or smooth objects (eg, beads, stones), foreign bodies positioned beyond the isthmus of the EAC or against the tympanic membrane (TM), nongraspable objects, and foreign bodies that have been present for more than 24 hours are less graspable, with lower rates of success and higher complication rates.[10–12] Instruments such as a right-angle hook, a Rosen needle, or a cerumen curette can be maneuvered between the foreign body and the EAC to pull the foreign body laterally. Balloon-tip catheters, including commercially available devices, such as the Katz extractor (InHealth Technologies, Carpinteria, CA, USA), function similarly by passing distally to the foreign body and allowing a laterally directed force to remove the object. A lasso can be fashioned using monofilament suture and a curette or other ring-tip instrument, such as a Jobson-Horne probe, and the suture can be passed around the foreign body and subsequently pulled out of the EAC.[8] Avoiding medially directed forces protects the TM and middle ear from further risk of damage.

Live insects present challenges beyond inert foreign bodies as they can move, causing trauma and quickly reducing patient comfort and compliance. Instillation of mineral oil or lidocaine into the EAC can quickly immobilize or kill the insect.[6,13,14] Filling the EAC with water can float the insect out of the canal or drown it.[15] After immobilization, the insect can then be removed similarly to other foreign bodies.

Micro suction can be used to remove friable material, particulate, and dead insects. The Schuknecht Foreign Body Remover (GYRUS ACMI, Bartlett, TN, USA) and the

Table 1
Instruments for external ear canal foreign body removal

Instrument	Advantages/Indications	Disadvantages/Contraindications
Micro alligator forceps Hartman foreign body forceps	Grasp thin objects or edges of objects Larger graspable objects	Not useful for large, round, firm objects that are unable to be grasped
Right angle ear hook Cerumen curette (eg, Buck, Shapleigh, Billeau) Rosen needle Suture lasso Balloon-tip catheter	Smooth, round, or other nongraspable objects	Placing metal instruments against the ear canal may be uncomfortable and increase risk of trauma to the ear canal skin or tympanic membrane in an uncooperative patient Placing instruments medial to foreign bodies may lead to blind manipulation
Micro suction (eg, Baron suction tubes)	Can easily remove particulate, debris, and small/light objects	
Magnetic probe	Magnetic or ferrous objects	
Irrigation	Useful for immobilizing/killing insects prior to removal and for small, loose objects. Easy to perform.	Contraindicated for removal of batteries on in patients with tympanic membrane perforations or unknown tympanic membrane status. Can cause organic material to swell.

VacuTIP Foreign Body Suction Tip (Summit Medical, St. Paul, MN, USA) are designed to augment metal suction tips with a flexible suction cup to conform to spherical objects. These, however, require the availability of a specific product. Irrigation can be used as an aid to suction by moistening the material, which then allows the suction to seal around the material to increase the force of the suction.

Adhesives may require treatment to remove their bond to the skin prior to removal. Solvents, including acetone and 3% hydrogen peroxide, can de-bond cyanoacrylate adhesive (sold commercially as Superglue, Power glue, and Instant glue).[16] Acetone has also been described in the removal of chewing gum[17] and to dissolve polystyrene.[18] More irritating or toxic solvents should be avoided.[19,20] Directed applications of chemical solutions can be used based on the chemical properties of a foreign body. For example, acidic Burow's solution (which contains aluminum acetate) has been used to dissolve cement in the EAC.[21] After using solvents, the EAC can then be cleansed with saline or water to remove any residual solvent.

Adhesive materials can adhere to nongraspable objects but can result in iatrogenic foreign bodies. A small amount of cyanoacrylate adhesive placed on the end of a swab stick has been described for removing beads and beans.[22] In another report, impression material (acrylic, dental alginate, silicone, and polysulfide) was placed into the EAC and allowed to cure. The impression material was then removed along with the foreign body. This technique may not be suitable for impacted foreign bodies. Patients with TM perforations are at risk of the impression material passing into the middle ear space.[23]

Expansile or semiliquid materials can produce additional challenges. The material may extend beyond the boundaries of the EAC in the presence of a TM perforation and become unreachable by a transcanal approach. Translocation of ear mold impression material into the middle ear can encase the ossicular chain and further spread into the Eustachian tube and mastoid cavity, potentially requiring surgical excision. A computed tomography (CT) scan can be useful in preoperative planning to evaluate the extent of a foreign body.[24,25]

For most EAC foreign bodies, there is low risk in deferring removal attempts for a brief period of time until experienced personnel and the appropriate instruments are available. Batteries, however, can cause liquefactive necrosis and require urgent removal.[26–28] A magnetic probe can be used to atraumatically remove batteries and ferrous foreign bodies.[29,30] A magnetic bridle nasal feeding tube retaining system kit (Applied Medical Technology, Inc, Brecksville, OH, USA) can be placed against the foreign body, and then the bridle and foreign body can be removed together.[4]

Operative management under local or general anesthesia

For some patients who undergo unsuccessful foreign body removal, re-examination at a later time with binocular otomicroscopy and microinstrumentation is appropriate. However, for patients who are uncooperative and unable to be immobilized or who cannot tolerate instrumentation, sedation or general anesthesia may be required. For an adult with medical comorbidities or the desire to avoid general anesthesia, lidocaine canal injections can provide local anesthesia. Rather than the traditional four-quadrant injection, canal injections in an awake patient are made by the first injection at 12 o'clock and then traveling shorter distances, alternating anterior and posterior injections, injecting where the local anesthetic has already anesthetized the soft tissue, until the entire circumference is anesthetized.

The operating room is set up similarly to performing myringotomy. After induction of general anesthesia, mask ventilation may be continued, or a laryngeal mask airway or endotracheal tube may be placed. The ear is then examined under binocular microscopy. A myringotomy tray containing a curette, alligator forceps, Rosen needle, and right angle is usually sufficient instrumentation for removal. Additional instrumentation can be supplemented as needed (reviewed in **Table 1**). Following removal, the ear is again examined for evidence of any damage to the ear canal, TM, or ossicular chain, and then the patient is awakened and taken to the recovery room.

DISCUSSION
Complications Related to Foreign Body

Complications may arise from the presence of the foreign body itself or from instrumentation during removal. Increased number of removal attempts and longer duration of foreign body impaction result in increased complication rates.[6] Aural foreign bodies may go unnoticed for a period of time until discovered on routine examination. By then, secondary infection may have occurred and present with inflammatory changes (marked by otorrhea and canal edema or granulation) unresponsive to medical treatment that only resolve with removing the nidus of infection.[5]

Some types of foreign bodies cause particular complications, most significantly button batteries, which should be removed urgently. Button batteries can cause injury due to either leakage of battery content, the primary cause of injury in alkaline batteries, or through generation of a current that hydrolyzes tissue fluids, producing hydroxide at the battery's negative pole. The latter is the source of injury for the more powerful lithium button batteries increasingly used in consumer electronics.[31] Alkaline burn injury due to liquefactive necrosis dissolves protein and collagen, saponifies lipids, and dehydrates tissue cells, causing damages that can mimic malignant otitis externa.[26,27] In the presence of a button battery, otic drops are absolutely contraindicated as their electrolyte solution can enhance corrosion of the crimp area of the battery, accelerating battery leakage.[32] In a review of 8 patients, button batteries in the ear caused TM perforation (n = 3) or total destruction (n = 3), marked canal skin dermal necrosis with exposed bone (n = 7), worsened hearing loss (n = 3), ossicular destruction (n = 2), and facial nerve paralysis with chondritis (n = 1).[32]

Molten metal or hot spark ("slag") ear injuries are uncommon but well known because of their tendency to create recalcitrant TM perforations and chronic otorrhea. Welders who work overhead in cramped conditions near other welders are particularly vulnerable and should wear flame-resistant ear plugs.[33] Slag can reach 1000°C, which can devascularize and destroy soft tissues with subsequent scarring, such that perforations may progressively enlarge over time. Slag can implant into the EAC or middle ear, causing a foreign body tissue reaction that promotes continued otorrhea, further complicating repair efforts and decreasing the likelihood of tympanoplasty success. Rarely, ossicular injury, facial nerve injury, peripheral vestibulopathy, and profound sensorineural hearing loss have occurred.[34–36] Various techniques have been described to improve tympanoplasty success, including removal of the imbedded foreign body, use of cartilage, silastic, and (of historic interest) tympanic homograft with intact malleus.[37,38]

Cotton buds dislodged from cotton-tipped applicators represent the most common aural foreign body in adults. Most often, these are removed with no to minimal sequelae. However, Woodley and colleagues described two patients who developed severe complications due to cotton buds impacted for prolonged periods. One developed a perichondritis that progressed to suppurative labyrinthitis with lateral semicircular canal fistula seen on CT. The second developed acute mastoiditis with cochlear fistula in the basal turn, temporomandibular joint erosion and postauricular gas formation. Both required operative management for debridement and removal of the foreign body in addition to medical management of the infection.[39] Charlton and colleagues described a healthy 31-year-old who developed necrotizing otitis externa due to a retained cotton bud, who presented with ipsilateral temporal subdural abscesses. He was managed with operative debridement of the EAC, cortical mastoidectomy, and prolonged intravenous antibiotic course.[40]

Complications Related to Removal

Published rates of success and complications during removal by an ED physician or otolaryngologist vary widely. Success rates in the ED setting range from 7% to 80%, with complication rates ranging from 1.5% to 47%.[10,41,42] Complications associated with removal include lacerations and bleeding in the EAC; less commonly, rupture of the TM or otitis externa; and rarely, ossicular disruption with hearing loss and vertigo.[43] Bressler and Shelton reported lower complication rates with initial otolaryngologist removal (6%) compared with prior attempts by the referring provider (67%).[6] Weksler and colleagues reported a similar rate of any complications following removal by pediatric emergency physicians (35.6%) versus otolaryngologists (26.8%, $P = .144$), but a very high rate of referral to otolaryngologists for the first attempt (77.8%).[44]

Irrigation is a preferred technique for EAC foreign body removal for some nonotolaryngologists; however, this method has several limitations.[45] High-pressure irrigation, such as from jet irrigation, can cause TM rupture, ossicular chain disruption, perilymph fistula, or subluxation of the stapedial footplate.[46] Cold irrigation can cause vertigo from the caloric effect. Hygroscopic foreign bodies, such as beans, peas, seeds, or other organic objects, can absorb moisture and swell.[47] Irrigation is contraindicated in patients with perforated TMs, or instances when the TM status is unknown.

Lidocaine is often instilled into the ear prior to insect removal. Though lidocaine quickly paralyzes an insect, sometimes it may cause the insect to rapidly move, inciting patient distress. Additionally, in the presence of a TM perforation, lidocaine may penetrate via the round window, causing inner ear symptoms including vertigo.[6,48,49] When vertigo occurs, it presents with a delayed onset of several minutes following the lidocaine exposure and persists for multiple hours. Mineral oil to drown the insect is a good alternative; however, this theoretically takes longer and may not be immediately available in the ED.[6]

SUMMARY

Foreign bodies in the EAC are a common presenting complaint to the ED. Instrumentation choice depends on the size, shape, and position of the foreign body. Irrigation should be avoided in the presence of hygroscopic organic matter, which may swell. Button batteries should be removed urgently, and otic drops and irrigation are strictly contraindicated. Otolaryngology consultation should be considered in patients with prior unsuccessful removal attempts, active canal inflammatory response and otorrhea, or patient intolerance of removal.

CLINICS CARE POINTS

- Forceps are useful for graspable objects and are often used by emergency physicians without referral to an otolaryngologist.
- Binocular microscopy with microinstrumentation, including angled hooks and currettes, is useful for hard, spherical objects, though general anesthesia may be required in an uncooperative patient.

- Remove button batteries urgently; otic drops and irrigation are strictly contraindicated.
- Douse live insects preferentially in mineral oil prior to removal, as lidocaine in the presence of a TM perforation can cause severe vertigo.

DISCLOSURE

The authors have no disclosures.

REFERENCES

1. Duan M, Morvil G, Badron J, et al. Epidemiological trends and outcomes of children with aural foreign bodies in Singapore. Ann Acad Med Singap 2022;51(6): 351–6.
2. Gold KR, Wester JL, Gold R. Foreign Body in External Ear Canal: An Unusual Cause of Chronic Cough. Am J Med 2017;130(4):e143–4.
3. Morris S, Osborne MS, McDermott AL. Will children ever learn? Removal of nasal and aural foreign bodies: A study of hospital episode statistics. Ann R Coll Surg Engl 2018;100(8):1–3.
4. Reyes-Chicuellar N, Crossland G. Extraction of Aural Foreign Bodies in a Rural Setting: 10-Year Review and a Novel Method to Remove Magnetic Stones. Ear Nose Throat J 2021. 1455613211006007.
5. Kim KH, Chung JH, Byun H, et al. Clinical Characteristics of External Auditory Canal Foreign Bodies in Children and Adolescents. Ear Nose Throat J 2020;99(10): 648–53.
6. Bressler K, Shelton C. Ear foreign-body removal a review of 98 consecutive cases. Laryngoscope 1993;103(4 Pt 1):367–70.
7. Kadish H. Ear and nose foreign bodies: "It is all about the tools". Clin Pediatr (Phila). 2005;44(8):665–70.
8. Ng TT. Aural foreign body removal: There is no one-size-fits-all method. Open Access Emerg Med 2018;10:177–82.
9. Morley HL. Iatrogenic foreign body in an adult with presbyacusis. BMJ Case Rep 2018;2018. bcr2017222913.
10. Dimuzio J, Deschler G. Emergency Department Management of Foreign Bodies of the External Auditory Canal in Children. Otol Neurotol 2002;23(4):473–5.
11. Schulze SL, Kerschner J, Beste D. Pediatric external auditory canal foreign bodies: A review of 698 cases. Otolaryngol Head Neck Surg 2002;127(1):73–8.
12. Thompson SK, Wein RO, Dutcher PO. External Auditory Canal Foreign Body Removal: Management Practices and Outcomes From the Division of Otolaryngology-Head and Neck Surgely Send Correspondence to. Laryngoscope 2003;113(11):1912–5.
13. Leffler S, Cheney P, Tandberg D. Chemical Immobilization and Killing of Intra-Aural Roaches: An In Vitro Comparative Study. Ann Emerg Med 1993;22(12):1795–8.
14. Antonelli PJ, Ahmadi A, Prevatt A. Insecticidal Activity of Common Reagents for Insect Foreign Bodies of the Ear. Laryngoscope 2001;111(1):15–20.
15. Kumar S. Management of foreign bodies in the ear, nose and throat. Emerg Med Australas 2004;16(1):17–20.
16. Dimitriadis P, Rourke T, Colquhoun-Flannery W, et al. 2013) Superglue ear our experience and a review of the literature. B-ENT 2013;9(4):325–8.
17. Chisholm EJ, Barber-Craig H, Farrell R. Chewing gum removal from the ear using acetone. J Laryngol Otol 2003;117(4):325.

18. White SJ, Broner S. The Use of Acetone to Dissolve a Styrofoam Impaction of the Ear. Ann Emerg Med 1994;23(3):580–2.
19. Picton-Robinson I. Danger of instant adhesives. Br Med J 1977;2(6086):581–2.
20. Persaud R. Short Communication A novel approach to the removal of superglue from the ear. J Laryngol Otol 2001;115(11):901–2.
21. Naoi Y, Kariya S, Tachibana T, et al. Application of Burow's solution for cement foreign body in the external auditory canal. Eur Ann Otorhinolaryngol Head Neck Dis 2019;136(5):397–9.
22. Pride H, Schwab R, Pride. (1989) A new technique for removing foreign bodies of the external auditory canal. Pediatr Emerg Care 1989;5(2):135–6.
23. Raz S, Newahk MA, Hildlng D. Impression materials for removal of aural foreign bodies. Ann Otol Rhinol Laryngol 1977;86(3 Pt 1):396–9.
24. Kohan D, Sorin A, Marra S, et al. Surgical Management of Complications after Hearing Aid Fitting. Laryngoscope 2004;114(2):317–22.
25. Jacob A, Morris TJ, Welling DB. Leaving a lasting impression: Ear mold impressions as middle ear foreign bodies. Ann Otol Rhinol Laryngol 2006;115(12):912–6.
26. Premachandra DJ, McRae D. Severe tissue destruction in the ear caused by alkaline button batteries. Postgrad Med J 1990;66(771):52–3.
27. Bhisitkul DM, Dunham M. An unsuspected alkaline battery foreign body presenting as malignant otitis externa. Pediatr Emerg Care 1992;8(3):141–2.
28. Thabet MH, Basha WM, Askar S. Button battery foreign bodies in children: Hazards, management, and recommendations. BioMed Res Int 2013;2013:846091.
29. Nivatvongs W, Ghabour M, Dhanasekar G. Difficult button battery ear foreign body removal: The magnetic solution. J Laryngol Otol 2015;129(1):93–4.
30. Scott RA, Wood C, Khan I. The novel use of a nasal bridle system to remove a foreign body in the ear. Clin Case Rep 2019;7(7):1439–41.
31. Litovitz T, Whitaker N, Clark L, et al. Emerging battery-ingestion hazard: Clinical implications. Pediatrics 2010;125(6):1168–77.
32. Kavanagh K, Litovitz T. Miniature battery foreign bodies in auditory and nasal cavities. JAMA 1986;255(11):1470–2. http://jama.jamanetwork.com/.
33. Simons JP, Eibling DE. Tympanic membrane perforation and retained metal slag after a welding injury. Otolaryngol Head Neck Surg 2005;133(4):635–6.
34. Panosian MS, Dutcher PO. Transtympanic facial nerve injury in welders. Occup Med (Lond) 1994;44(2):99–101.
35. Stage J, Vinding T. Metal spark perforation of the tympanic membrane with deafness and facial paralysis. J Laryngol Otol 1986;100(6):699–700.
36. Eleftheriadou A, Chalastras T, Kyrmizakis D, et al. Metallic foreign body in middle ear: An unusual cause of hearing loss. Head Face Med 2007;3:23.
37. Keogh IJ, Portmann D. Drop weld thermal injuries to the middle ear. Rev Laryngol Otol Rhinol 2009;130(4–5):317–9.
38. Lesinski SG. Homograft (allograft) tympanoplasty update. Laryngoscope 1986;96(11):1211–20.
39. Woodley N, Mohd Slim MA, Tikka T, et al. Not "just" a foreign body in the ear canal. BMJ Case Rep 2019;12(4):e229302.
40. Charlton A, Janjua N, Rejali D. Cotton bud in external ear canal causing necrotising otitis externa and subdural abscess. BMJ Case Rep 2019;12(3):e227971.
41. Baker M. Foreign bodies of the ears and nose in childhood. Pediatr Emerg Care 1987;3(2):67–70.

42. Mackle T, Conlon B. Foreign bodies of the nose and ears in children: Should these be managed in the accident and emergency setting? Int J Pediatr Otorhinolaryngol 2006;70(3):425–8.
43. Kim A, Dean C, Parisier S. Injuries and foreign bodies of the external auditory canal. In: Bluestone C, Simons J, Healy G, editors. Bluestone and stool's pediatric otolaryngology. 5th edition. People's Medical Publishing House-USA; 2014. p. 880–1.
44. Weksler CW, Heiman E, Weiser G. Removal of external auditory canal foreign bodies in the pediatric emergency department - A retrospective comparison study. Int J Pediatr Otorhinolaryngol 2022;160:111247.
45. Fritz S, Kelen GD, Sivertson KT. Foreign bodies of the external auditory canal. Emerg Med Clin North Am 1987;5(2):183–92.
46. Dinsdale R, Roland P, Manning S, et al. Catastrophic otologic injury from oral jet irrigation of the external auditory canal. Laryngoscope 1991;101(1 Pt 1):75–8.
47. Brown J. Hydroscopic Properties of Organic Objects That May Present as Aural Foreign Bodies. J Clin Med Res 2010;2(4):172–6.
48. Cantrell H. More on removing cockroaches from the auditory canal. N Engl J Med 1986;314(11):720.
49. Simmons FB, Glattke TJ, Downie DB. Lidocaine in the Middle Ear A Unique Cause of Vertigo. Arch Otolaryngol 1973;98(1):42–3.

An Overview of Acute Otitis Externa

Ann Woodhouse Plum, MD*, Michele Wong, MD

KEYWORDS

- Acute otitis externa • Bacterial • Otalgia • Ear • Infection

KEY POINTS

- The pathogenesis of acute otitis externa is multifactorial and includes processes that traumatize the external auditory canal and initiate the process of inflammation, bacterial invasion, alteration of the microbial flora, and bacterial overgrowth.
- The most common presenting symptoms are otalgia, pruritus, and aural fullness.
- The topical antimicrobials are the first-line therapy for uncomplicated acute otitis media.

EPIDEMIOLOGY

Acute otitis externa (AOE), also known as "swimmer's ear," continues to represent the most common waterborne disease in the United States: In 2021, the Centers of Disease Control and Prevention estimated that otitis externa accounts for an annual 567,000 emergency department visits, 23,200 hospital admissions, and $564,000,000 total annual direct health care costs.[1] Most infections occur during summer months, 80% of cases in a large scale study, and the incidence of disease appears to be evenly distributed throughout age groups with the exception of a peak in the 7 to 12 age group and a decline in individuals aged 50 years or older.[2]

PATHOGENESIS/RISK FACTORS

The pathogenesis of AOE is multifactorial and includes processes that traumatize the external auditory canal (EAC) and initiate the process of inflammation, bacterial invasion, alteration of the microbial flora, and bacterial overgrowth. Factors that are associated with bacterial AOE include persistent moisture of the ear canal, trauma, ear plug or hearing aid usage, history of radiation therapy, immunocompromised state, high cerumen burden, which can promote water retention, foreign bodies, and dermatologic conditions such as seborrheic dermatitis.[3,4]

Department of Otolaryngology, State of New York Downstate Medical Center, 450 Clarkson Avenue, MSC 126, Brooklyn NY 11203, USA
* Corresponding author.
E-mail address: ann.plum@downstate.edu

Otolaryngol Clin N Am 56 (2023) 891–896
https://doi.org/10.1016/j.otc.2023.06.006
0030-6665/23/© 2023 Elsevier Inc. All rights reserved.

MICROBIOLOGY

AOE can be due to bacterial or fungal pathogens. Studies stemming from the significant incidence of AOE among military personnel during World War II clarified the etiology of AOE as being predominantly bacterial rather than fungal.[5,6] Primary infection with fungi is less common in AOE and can occur as a co-pathogen with bacteria, particularly in immunocompromised patients or following a prolonged course of topical antibiotics to the EAC. *Aspergillus* and *Candida* species are the most common fungal pathogens.[2,3] Acute fungal otitis externa is a complex and nuanced topic and will be covered in a different chapter. In North America, nearly 98% of all AOE has a bacterial etiology.[2] Early culture-based studies in the mid-1900s identified *Pseudomonas* as the primary pathogen in AOE, which has been further confirmed in subsequent large- and small-scale phenotypic and genotypic investigations in the early 2000s.[2,7] The most frequently isolated organism in AOE is predominantly *Pseudomonas aeruginosa* (38%), followed by *Staphylococcus epidermidis* (9.7%) and *Staphylococcus aureus* (7.8%).[2]

Advances in laboratory techniques and increasing interest in human microbiome studies have led to increasing data on the microbiome of the EAC in healthy individuals.[8,9] Rough trends have emerged from recent small-scale studies: Healthy EACs have higher microbiome diversity than those with otitis externa.[8,10,11] The most common bacteria in the microbiome of healthy EACs studied include *Staphylococcus auricularis*, *Propionibacterium acnes*, *Alloiococcus otitis*, *Turicella otitidis*, and *Corynebacterium otitidis*.[8,9] These studies suggest there may be therapeutic potential in modulating the EAC microbiome and that the natural flora present in an individual's EAC may be an important factor in the development of AOE although much remains to be elucidated.[8,9]

DIAGNOSIS

The diagnosis of AOE is a clinical one.

History and Physical Examination

Patients typically present with rapid onset of symptoms, which is typically less than 48 hours, and signs associated with inflammation of the affected ear canal.[3] The most common presenting symptoms are otalgia, pruritus, and aural fullness.[3] The otalgia may be exacerbated by manipulation of the tragus or pinna or movement of the temporomandibular joint.[3] These symptoms may be associated with or without hearing loss or otorrhea.[3] Patients may present with auricular cellulitis or lymphadenopathy.[3,12]

Otoscopy/Otomicroscopy

In acute bacterial otitis externa, the EAC is often edematous and erythematous.[3] Edema of the ear canal may prevent visualization of the tympanic membrane (TM) in severe cases. Otorrhea or debris of the canal may also be seen. When visualized, the appearance of the TM in bacterial AOE may be erythematous and similar in appearance to acute otitis media (AOM).[3] Evidence of tympanostomy tubes or a nonintact TM should be noted as their presence can significantly change management and may suggest an otitis media with a spontaneous rupture of the TM or tube otorrhea.[3] Fungal otitis externa (primary or secondary) should be suspected if exudates with white filamentous hyphae or black spores are visualized, best seen with otomicroscopy.[3,4] Malignant otitis externa or malignancy should be considered if granulation tissue is noted in the EAC.[3] A canal cholesteatoma or keratitis obturans should be considered if there is buildup of keratinaceous debris with erosion or expansion of the boney walls of the EAC.

Tympanometry/Pneumatic Otoscopy

Pneumatic otoscopy or tympanometry may be used to aid in diagnosis and would reveal preserved mobility of the TM in AOE and normal tympanometry (Type A).[3] However, significant canal edema or the presence of significant debris or otorrhea may affect the tympanometry results in the case of AOE. Pneumatic otoscopy would reveal no mobility or limited mobility of the TM for a patient affected by AOM with or without a perforation or in the case of tube otorrhea, and tympanometry would be consistent with a type B tympanogram with either a normal or large canal volume.

Culture

A culture of the ear canal may be performed and can be useful in cases where a patient fails to respond to treatment to evaluate for alternative causes of infection such as bacteria with antibiotic resistance, fungi, or unusual causes of infection.[3,13]

Imaging

In most cases of AOE, imaging is not required. Imaging may be performed in patients with suspected necrotizing (malignant) otitis externa or in the management of underlying middle-ear disease.[14,15] Malignant otitis externa is a rare but potentially fatal disorder in which cellulitis of the EAC progressed into osteomyelitis which can involve the skull base.[3] Elderly, diabetic, and immunocompromised patients are specifically at risk for this.[3] The presentation of necrotizing otitis externa typically includes severe, chronic otalgia, otorrhea, and cranial nerve (CN) deficits of CN VII to XII.[14] The management of this disorder is beyond the scope of the present discussion.

Differential Diagnosis

Fungal otitis externa
Malignant otitis externa
Dermatitis
Keratosis obturans
Ceruminosis obturans
Canal cholesteatoma

MANAGEMENT

The management of bacterial AOE centers on analgesia, treating the underlying bacterial infection and preventing recurrence. The signs and symptoms of uncomplicated AOE typically improve within 48 to 72 hours of initiating appropriate treatment.[3] Patients with suspected AOE who do not improve within this timeframe should be clinically re-evaluated.[3]

Analgesia

The pain from bacterial AOE can be severe due to the robust innervation of the ear; therefore, the severity of pain should be assessed.[3,16] Oral agents for analgesia such as acetaminophen or nonsteroidal anti-inflammatory drugs typically provide relief of mild to moderate pain.[3,16] The appropriate dosing and frequency (as needed versus scheduled) are guided by understanding that preventing pain is simpler than treating pain. In the case of procedure-related pain control and control of severe pain, opioids may be considered in select patients.[3] Topical anesthetic ear drops may be considered but can also mask the progression of the underlying disease and should not be used in patients with a nonintact TM due to potential ototoxicity.[3] Likewise, the addition of a topical steroid may also improve pain control.[3]

Antimicrobial Therapy

The use of systemic antibiotics (oral or parenteral) for initial treatment of uncomplicated bacterial AOE is strongly discouraged.[3,16] The use of systemic antibiotic therapy is associated with significant harms, the most consequential of which is the development of bacterial resistance.[17]

Topical preparations of antimicrobial therapy are recommended as the first-line therapy in bacterial AOE by American Academy of Otolaryngology- Head and Neck Surgery clinical practice guidelines for their safety and efficacy in randomized trials.[3,16] Topical delivery allows for the delivery of significantly higher concentrations of antimicrobials directly to infected tissue.[3] Ototopical therapy should be initiated for a minimum of 7 days.[3] However, caution should be taken not to prolong treatment and cause a fungal otitis externa due to alterations of the normal flora.[3] Patients with persistent symptoms beyond 7 days should be re-evaluated.[3]

Based on AAO-HNS clinical practice guidelines, selection of topical antimicrobial preparations may be based on patient preference and clinician experience due to no significant difference in efficacy between most topical antimicrobial and steroid preparations in patients with uncomplicated bacterial AOE and an intact TM.[3] Topical antibiotic preparations may include an aminoglycoside, polymyxin B, and/or a quinolone.[3] Steroid therapy, such as hydrocortisone or dexamethasone, may be added to the antimicrobial therapy to help with analgesia and canal edema.[3] Finally, a low-pH antiseptic such as acetic acid may be considered.[3]

Special consideration for patients with a known or suspected nonintact TM is advised when selecting a topical antimicrobial therapy.[3] Ototoxic substances or those with ototoxic potential must be avoided in these patients. Aminoglycosides, topical drops that contain alcohol or have a low pH, should be avoided in patients with a nonintact TM because of the risk of ototoxic injury to the structures of the middle ear and potential for permanent sensorineural hearing loss.[3]

Enhancing Treatment Delivery

Both aural toilet and placement of an ear canal wick can enhance delivery of topical antimicrobial drops in an obstructed ear canal. Aural toilet should be considered as this allows the topical antimicrobials to directly contact the areas of cellulitis.[3] In cases of severe canal edema, the placement of an ear wick promotes delivery of antimicrobial drops through the length of the canal.

Ototopical drug delivery to the ear may be hindered due to poor adherence or ineffective self-administration, which can lead to undertreatment. Clear explanation of instructions by the clinician is necessary to address these barriers. Antimicrobial drops should be administered with the patient lying down and the affected ear facing upward until the drops pass into the canal.[3] Gentle movement of the pinna or palpation of the tragus may promote delivery of the drops medially down the canal.[3] In addition, having another person apply the drops enhances compliance with the treatment regimen.[3]

Special Considerations

Supplemental treatment with systemic antibiotics in addition to topical therapy is recommended in specific circumstances. In regards to disease factors, the addition of systemic antimicrobials should occur if there is extension outside the EAC or if there is an obstruction that cannot be completely removed from the EAC that may prevent complete delivery of topical therapy.[3,15] In terms of patient factors, systemic therapy should be added if patients are unable to comply with topical therapy, there is a history of diabetes, or in patients with an impaired immune system.[3,15] Systemic antibiotics should be directed against *Pseudomonas* and *Staphylococcus*.[3]

Monitoring

Complete clinical resolution of bacterial AOE may take up to 2 weeks.[3] Patients who do not respond to initial therapy within 48 to 72 hours should be re-evaluated.[3] Patients should be asked about issues with treatment adherence or delivery in addition to assessing for clinical resolution.[3] Reassessment allows for determining if aural toilet, placement of an ear wick, changes to pain management and antibiotic therapy, and considering alternative diagnoses are appropriate.[3]

Prevention

Strategies at preventing bacterial AOE are patient specific but can be necessary in cases where there is recurrence. These strategies may include limiting water exposure, moisture retention of the ear canal, managing recurrent cerumen impaction, and minimizing trauma to the ear canal.[3,4,15] Trauma can be secondary to self-cleaning of the ear canal with cotton-tipped swabs, foreign bodies, and use of hearing aids.[3,4,15] During treatment of AOE, patients should avoid manipulating the ear, and water restrictions should be discussed.[3]

SUMMARY

The diagnosis of bacterial AOE is largely clinical and characteristically presents with rapid onset of symptoms and signs associated with inflammation of the affected ear canal. The most common presenting symptoms are otalgia, pruritus, and aural fullness. The management of AOE centers on analgesia, treating the underlying infection and preventing recurrence. The topical antimicrobials are the first-line therapy for uncomplicated AOM. Complete clinical resolution of bacterial AOE may take up to 2 weeks. Patients who do not respond to the initial therapy within 48 to 72 hours should be re-evaluated.

CLINICS CARE POINTS

- Aural toilet can be a helpful tool in the treatment of acute otitis externa and should be strongly considered.
- While topical antimicrobials are the cornerstone of treatment, in an uncooperative patient or one with severe or complicated disease, systemic antimicrobials can be considered.
- One should always consider preventative measures in the case of patients with recurrent episodes of acute otitis externa.

DISCLOSURE

The authors have nothing to disclose.

REFERENCES

1. Collier SA, Deng L, Adam EA, et al. Estimate of burden and direct healthcare cost of infectious waterborne disease in the United States. Emerg Infect Dis 2021;27(1):140.

2. Roland PS, Stroman DW. Microbiology of acute otitis externa. Laryngoscope 2002;112(7):1166–77.
3. Rosenfeld RM, Schwartz SR, Cannon CR, et al. Clinical practice guideline: acute otitis externa. Otolaryngology-Head Neck Surg (Tokyo) 2014;150:S1–24.
4. Hirsch BE. Infections of the external ear. Am J Otolaryngol 1992;13(3):145–55.
5. Nelson RF. External otitis in the South Pacific. Ann Otol Rhinol Laryngol 1945; 54(2):367–72.
6. Singer DE, Freeman E, Hoffert WR, et al. XXIV Otitis Externa: Bacteriological and Mycological Studies. Ann Otol Rhinol Laryngol 1952;61(2):317–30.
7. Senturia BH. Etiology of external otitis. Laryngoscope 1945;55(6):277–93.
8. Frank DN, Spiegelman GB, Davis W, et al. Culture-independent molecular analysis of microbial constituents of the healthy human outer ear. J Clin Microbiol 2003;41(1):295–303.
9. Sjövall A, Aho VT, Hyyrynen T, et al. Microbiome of the healthy external auditory canal. Otol Neurotol 2021;42(5):e609–14.
10. Kim SK, Han SJ, Hong SJ, et al. Microbiome of Acute Otitis Externa. J Clin Med 2022;11(23):7074.
11. Lee JS, Lee SM, Son HS, et al. Analysis of the Microbiome of the Ear Canal in Normal Individuals and Patients with Chronic Otitis Externa. Ann Dermatol 2022;34(6):461–71.
12. Lucente FE, Lawson W, Novick NL. The external ear. Philadelphia, PA: WB Saunders Company; 1995.
13. Saunders JE, Raju RP, Boone JL, et al. Antibiotic resistance and otomycosis in the draining ear: culture results by diagnosis. Am J Otolaryngol 2011;32(6):470–6.
14. Grandis JR, Curtin HD, Yu VL. Necrotizing (malignant) external otitis: prospective comparison of CT and MR imaging in diagnosis and follow-up. Radiology 1995; 196(2):499–504.
15. Ruckenstein MJ. Infections of the external ear. In: Cummings otolaryngology: head & neck surgery. 7th edition. Philadelphia, PA: Mosby; 2021. p. 2093–100.e2.
16. Bhattacharyya N, Kepnes LJ. Initial impact of the acute otitis externa clinical practice guideline on clinical care. Otolaryngology-Head Neck Surg (Tokyo) 2011;145(3):414–7.
17. Dibb WL. Microbial aetiology of otitis externa. J Infect 1991;22(3):233–9.

External Ear Disease
Keratinaceous Lesions of the External Auditory Canal

Tina Munjal, MD, Peter J. Kullar, MA, PhD, FRCS,
Jennifer Alyono, MD, MS*

KEYWORDS

- Keratinaceous lesions • External auditory canal cholesteatoma • Keratosis obturans

KEY POINTS

- Keratosis obturans is classically defined by the overaccumulation of keratin debris in the external auditory canal, leading to hearing loss and severe, acute otalgia.
- External auditory canal cholesteatoma is classically defined by localized invasion of squamous epithelium causing osteonecrosis of the underlying bone, leading to otorrhea and chronic, dull otalgia.
- Keratosis obturans is defined as silent or inflammatory. External auditory canal cholesteatoma may be categorized as primary idiopathic, or secondary to an underlying cause (congenital, posttraumatic, iatrogenic, postobstructive, and/or postinflammatory).
- While both pathologies often respond well to in-clinic debridement, surgery may be required for more extensive disease. While surgery is more likely to be required for external auditory canal cholesteatoma than it is for keratosis obturans, the approaches to each pathology are similar.

INTRODUCTION

The external auditory canal (EAC) skin consists of keratinizing stratified squamous epithelium and is in continuity with the epithelium of the tympanic membrane.[1] In this article, we review two keratinaceous lesions affecting the EAC: keratosis obturans (KO) and EAC cholesteatoma (EACC). Historically, these two lesions were considered to be the same process, and the terms were used interchangeably. In 1850, Toynbee described a lesion of the EAC consisting of epidermal scales which he called "specimens of molluscum contagiosum."[2] To this day, there is disagreement in the literature as to whether this original description was of KO or EACC. Modern imaging and

Department of Otolaryngology – Head & Neck Surgery, Stanford University School of Medicine, 801 Welch Road, Palo Alto, CA 94304, USA
* Corresponding author.
E-mail address: jalyono@stanford.edu

Otolaryngol Clin N Am 56 (2023) 897–908
https://doi.org/10.1016/j.otc.2023.06.013
0030-6665/23/© 2023 Elsevier Inc. All rights reserved.

oto.theclinics.com

histopathologic analytic techniques have proven these to be 2 discrete but similar entities. Herein we review the diagnosis, pathophysiology, and management of each.

KERATOSIS OBTURANS
Definitions, Signs, and Symptoms

KO is a condition characterized by the overaccumulation of keratin, a structural fibrous protein found in the skin, hair, and nails, in the external auditory canal. KO is defined by the presence of an obstructive plug of desquamated keratin within a dilated external auditory meatus, associated with a thickened tympanic membrane.[3,4] Important differential diagnoses include external auditory canal cholesteatoma and skull base osteomyelitis. Until the 19th century KO and EACC were considered the same condition until they were differentiated by Piepergerdes. In this seminal article, KO was defined as the deposition of large plugs of desquamated keratin in a widened ear canal and EACC as the invasion of squamous tissue into a focal area of eroded ear canal.[4] Although the canal wall is involved in both conditions, in KO the ear canal is widened by the circumferential involvement of bone, whereas in EACC there is focal bony erosion, frequently in the posteroinferior ear canal.

KO typically presents in young adults and may develop in previously normal ear canals. The most consistent symptoms of KO are significant otalgia and a progressive conductive hearing loss. Additionally, keratinous obstruction of the canal may impede the ear's self-cleaning mechanism and increase the risk of infection.[5,6] The condition is typically unilateral but may also be bilateral in 44% of patients.[7] The incidence has been estimated at 4-5 patients per 1000 otology patients and has been reported as more common in females than males.[8] There have been historical associations with sinusitis and bronchiectasis; however, this is not represented in modern case series.[6,9–11]

Pathophysiology and Risk Factors

Although KO has been associated with skin conditions including seborrheic dermatitis and eczema, the underlying pathological mechanisms are yet to be fully determined. It is thought that KO results from the aberrant epithelial migration of the ear canal skin. It has been shown in one patient with KO that epithelial migration was restricted in the inferior quadrant of the tympanic membrane due to areas of abnormal desquamation.[12] In a separate study in a patient with KO, the epithelium over the pars flaccida was shown to migrate towards the pars tensa (contrary to the normal physiologic direction of migration) and then inferiorly across the tympanic membrane.[13]

Impacted keratin acts as a nidus for infection and cultures from KO are typically polymicrobial with *Staphylococcus aureus* being the most commonly cultured organism. *Proteus mirabilis*, *Staphylococcus epidermidis*, *Klebsiella pneumoniae* and *Streptococci* are also found, whereas *Pseudomonas* is seldom isolated.[14]

It has been proposed that there are two types of KO: silent and inflammatory. The inflammatory type results from an acute bacterial or viral infection that leads to dysfunctional epithelial migration and the accumulation of a keratinous plug which resolves after removal. The silent type is not triggered by an infection and requires multiple removals.[14] Patients with the silent type require lifelong periodic ear cleaning due to the lack of normal migratory mechanism of the canal skin.[9]

Risk factors for KO include a history of seborrheic dermatitis, furunculosis, trauma particularly from the use of cotton buds, eczema, sympathetic stimulation of the cerumen glands, and tropical weather.[8,9]

Workup

Diagnosis is primarily made by history and microscopic examination of the ear. Typically, the diagnosis will be reached after several failed attempts to remove the plug from the canal. **Fig. 1** demonstrates an example of a keratin plug removed from the ear canal in a patient with keratosis obturans. On removal of the keratinous plug, it is noted to have a silvery-white matrix at the periphery. Removal of the matrix may result in bleeding due to neovascularization.[8] The canal may initially appear narrowed due to edema and granulation tissue which resolves on removal of the plug. This may reveal the annulus of the tympanic membrane "suspended in air" within a dilated but typically uneroded bony canal. CT imaging of the temporal bone is a useful adjunct in the diagnosis and important to aid surgical planning. Audiology is important to ascertain the degree of conductive hearing loss.

Tissue biopsy and histological examination is warranted if there is diagnostic uncertainty or if there is granulation tissue present in the EAC. In this case, apart from EACC, the differential diagnosis also includes ear canal squamous cell carcinoma, skull base osteomyelitis, and benign neoplasm with secondary infection.

Imaging

CT imaging of KO reveals a widened canal occluded by a well-defined soft tissue plug typically without bony erosion.[15] An example of this can be seen in **Fig. 2**. Axial CT of the head demonstrates circumferential widening of the right bony EAC with a layered plug of debris within the canal. There is notable absence of focal bony erosion. CT imaging is useful to exclude other diagnoses such as middle ear cholesteatoma and involvement of surrounding structures such as the facial nerve, middle and inner ear and the temporomandibular joint.[16]

Pathology

Histological examination of KO reveals an associated hyperplasia of the underlying epithelium with keratinized squames in a lamellar pattern and chronic inflammation within the subepithelial tissue, without evidence of erosion or necrosis of the bone of the external auditory canal.[3] In KO, keratin is deposited circumferentially resulting in a lamellar arrangement. This contrasts with EACC in which keratin is deposited from the sac randomly in all directions.[3] Unlike in EACC, in which immunostaining for EGFR and TGF-alpha are stronger than normal auditory canal skin, in KO there is no staining for these growth factors.[17]

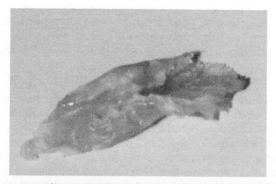

Fig. 1. *Clinical appearance of keratosis obturans.* Keratin plug after removal from the ear canal. (*From* Yael Raz, Chapter 110 - Keratosis Obturans and Canal Cholesteatoma, in Eugene N. Myers et al. Operative Otolaryngology: Head and Neck Surgery, Two-Volume Set, 2nd Edition. © 2008 by Saunders, an imprint of Elsevier Inc.)

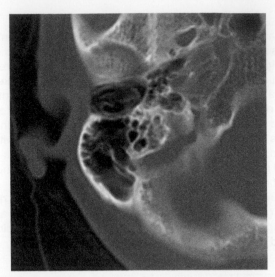

Fig. 2. *Imaging appearance of keratosis obturans.* Noncontrasted computed tomography of the head (right ear, axial section) demonstrating a layering plug of debris within the external auditory canal. There is circumferential widening of the canal wall but no focal bony erosion.

Treatment

The treatment for KO depends on the severity of the symptoms and the extent of keratin accumulation. In some cases, the condition may resolve without treatment, but in the majority of cases, mechanical removal of the keratin plug is required to reduce pain, improve hearing and prevent potential complications. Typically, this is performed in the office without the need for general anesthesia. Otic drops including hydrogen peroxide, mineral oil, and corticosteroids have been recommended to soften the plug before removal.[18] Topical treatment with antibiotic/steroid ear drops may have a short-term improvement but have not been demonstrated to achieve long term remission. A recent report suggested 57% of patients treated with topical miconazole/triamcinolone 0.1% cream had disease resolution. Miconazole is proposed to have a dual effect as an anti-fungal and reducing the hyperproliferative activity of keratinocytes. Triamcinolone is an anti-inflammatory and immunosuppressive corticosteroid with activity against the subepithelial inflammation.[19] In severe cases, canalplasty with split thickness skin grafting has been proposed; however, as skin grafts do not restore the normal migratory pathways of the ear canal, regular aural cleaning is often still required.[20]

Complications

Most cases of KO are confined to the ear canal, as classically there is no bony erosion. However, there are reports in the literature of extensive KO leading to both intra- and extratemporal complications. There have been no reports of intracranial complications.[14] Bony remodeling may result from the secretion of proteolytic enzymes or from pressure necrosis from the expanding keratin plug. This presumed bony erosion (not present in classical descriptions of KO) can lead to the involvement of the facial nerve in the mastoid and tympanic segments which may lead to a facial nerve palsy.[21] Other significant complications may result from the spread of KO into the temporomandibular joint, and middle and inner ear via the tympanic membrane, including labyrinthine fistula, dehiscence of the tegmen tympani, and sensorineural hearing loss.[22] Saunders and colleagues, describe a case of advanced KO with erosion of the temporomandibular joint and jugular bulb. In this case there was extensive erosion of the bony canal including automastoidectomy. This was managed surgically by formalizing the mastoidectomy and performing a large meatoplasty enabling post-operative mastoid cleaning.[22] However, in many of these reported cases of advanced KO with complications, it is not clear whether these represent the extreme of KO versus misclassified EACC.

EXTERNAL AUDITORY CANAL CHOLESTEATOMA
Definitions, Signs, and Symptoms

The term cholesteatoma describes a cyst lined with stratified squamous epithelium,[23] classically affecting the middle ear and mastoid. EAC cholesteatoma, or EACC, is a rare entity, affecting only 0.1-0.5% of otologic patients.[24] The signs and symptoms of EACC have considerable overlap with other canal pathologies, especially KO. EACC can be associated with otorrhea and chronic, unilateral dull pain on account of localized invasion of squamous epithelium, with associated osteonecrosis or bony sequestration.[4] The dull pain is thought to be due to the periosteitis.[25] Typically, the middle ear is normal in EACC, unlike in acquired epitympanic or mesotympanic cholesteatoma, and may remain clear if the disease remains limited to the canal. The tympanic membrane in KO may be thickened. However, the TM tends to appear normal in EACC.[3,4] Hearing loss due to the obstruction of the canal alone from EACC is relatively rare.[4] On the other hand, KO presents more with hearing loss and severe, acute pain on account of the large plugs of desquamated keratin in the EAC that cause overall widening of the bone of the EAC.[4,26]

KO tends to affect a younger demographic and a significant number of patients have bilateral disease. In contrast, primary idiopathic EACC is classically a disease of older adults with unilateral presentation.[4,7] Secondary EACC—a sequela of other otologic pathology—can affect any age group including pediatric patients.

Pathophysiology and Risk Factors

There are many underlying proposed mechanisms for the development of EACC. EACC can be categorized as primary, i.e., spontaneous, or secondary based on several underlying etiologies. The categories can be described as follows, based on a combination of clinical history, physical examination, and imaging characteristics.[27–29] Of note, in all of these, a key distinguishing feature of EACC regardless of etiologic categorization is the osteonecrosis and epithelial loss that are typically absent in KO.[25]

- Primary/Spontaneous (ie, Idiopathic): The patient has no prior history of ear disease, trauma, or surgery. On examination, there is well localized bony erosion in the inferior and posterior canal, just lateral to the annulus. In adults, spontaneous EACC always involves the floor of EAC and may also involve the posterior and anterior walls.[30] **Fig. 3** demonstrates the classic appearance of EACC on physical examination. Endoscopy in this patient shows a normal tympanic membrane medially, with evidence of squamous debris invaginating into the floor of the bony canal wall, leading to epithelial loss and underlying bony erosion. In pediatric patients, there appears be a predilection for the posterior canal wall.[31,32]
- Secondary
  - Congenital: This can occur in the setting of existing congenital stenosis of the EAC. Imaging demonstrates cholesteatoma medial to the stenosis with a possible atresia plate separating the EACC from the middle ear. 20% of

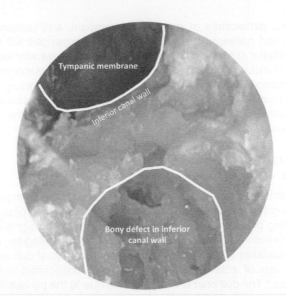

Fig. 3. *Clinical appearance of external auditory canal cholesteatoma.* Endoscopic image demonstrating normal tympanic membrane, with squamous debris and focal bony erosion of the inferior bony canal wall.

patients with congenital aural stenosis develop EACC, with female sex being a risk factor.[33] Prenatal isotretinoin exposure has also been linked to EACC, in the setting of EAC stenosis.[34]

- Posttraumatic: This can occur in a patient with a history of trauma, such as either a temporal bone fracture or penetrating injury of the EAC. The trauma may lead to acquired stenosis of the EAC or otherwise implantation of epithelium into an otherwise well aerated mastoid. There is typically a shorter time interval between injury and diagnosis for post-traumatic canal cholesteatoma relative to post-traumatic cholesteatoma of the attic and mastoid.[35]
- Iatrogenic
  - Postsurgical: The patient has a history of prior tympanomastoid surgery. Skin can invaginate through a defect in the posterior canal wall. EACC can also develop anteriorly due to blunting following lateral graft tympanoplasty. Small, limited keratin pearls are usually not considered EACC.
  - Postradiation: The patient has a history of radiation, with resulting soft tissue and bony changes.[36,37]
- Postobstructive: The patient has a history of occlusion of the EAC from causes such as osteoma, fibrous dysplasia, or foreign body.
- Postinflammatory: The patient has a history of chronic otitis externa.

Normal EAC skin demonstrates epithelial migration in a direction which coincides with the blood vessels supplying the epidermal layer of the tympanic membrane. In spontaneous EACC, however, there is a possible slowing of the migratory rate and desquamation, with complete absence of migration at the extreme.[38] One possibility is that the older demographic prone to spontaneous EACC has a poor blood supply of the EAC and tympanic membrane causing disruption in epithelial migration.[38] This is controversial, however, as a more recent study demonstrated that ears with EACC have normal migration except directly on crust-covered lesions.[30] Thus, the extent to which aberrant epithelial migration contributes to EACC is not fully elucidated (while aberrant epithelial migration *is* thought to contribute to KO[12]). Another possibility for the pathogenesis of EACC is the accumulation of keratin debris leading to changes in cellular proliferation within the EAC.[39] It has also been suggested that an initial focus of periosteitis is the cause of EACC rather than the consequence.[3] In pediatric spontaneous EACC, the proposed mechanism is repeated minor trauma to the EAC, such as through cotton bud use or habitual ear picking. Further, a possible predominance for right-sided EACC in pediatric patients also supports this hypothesis.[40] Risk factors for spontaneous EACC include advanced age, history of cotton bud use, hemodialysis, and diabetes mellitus.[41] Chronic bronchitis, congenital syphilis, and scarlet fever have also been linked with the formation of EACC.[26]

More than one underlying etiology is also possible, such as in the case of EACC due to underlying type I branchial cleft anomaly, which can be considered secondary to congenital, postobstructive, and postinflammatory causes.[42]

Workup

Diagnosis of EACC relies on the patient history and physical examination, with imaging serving as a useful adjunct in ascertaining the extent of disease for treatment planning. Tissue diagnosis is not typically required to make the diagnosis unless there is uncertainty. For both KO and EACC, the clinical examination is of utmost importance.

Imaging

If the depth of the cholesteatoma pocket cannot be visualized in the clinic with binocular microscopy, imaging of EACC is useful in determining extension into surrounding structures, such as the middle ear, mastoid, fallopian canal, and tegmen. On magnetic resonance imaging (MRI), the lesion will demonstrate diffusion restriction.[43] On computed tomography (CT), EACC appears as a hypoattenuating mass with bony erosion and may have intralesional bone fragments.[43] Shin and colleagues,[44] describe an imaging classification based on CT which can be useful for treatment planning, as later in discussion.

- Stage I: Disease is limited to the EAC.
- Stage II: Disease invades the tympanic membrane and middle ear.
- Stage III: Disease creates a defect of the EAC and involves mastoid air cells.
- Stage IV: Disease is beyond the temporal bone and may involve the glenoid or middle fossa.

From a differential diagnosis standpoint, often the history and examination will distinguish this pathology from others, though imaging can provide additional insight. KO demonstrates canal expansion typically in the absence of bony erosion or intralesional bone fragments. Medial canal fibrosis also does not demonstrate bony erosion. While skull base osteomyelitis can have bony erosion, it is also associated with fat infiltration, soft tissue swelling, and deep, unremitting pain.[45] Technetium-99m or citrate gallium-67 single photon emission CT (SPECT), as well as microbiologic studies, can further be useful in differentiating skull base osteomyelitis from EACC if the clinical picture is unclear.[25,46] **Fig. 4** demonstrates the imaging appearance of advanced EACC, with the involvement of (A) the posterior bony canal wall into the mastoid air cells, as well as (B) erosion into critical structures of the middle ear and mastoid including the incus and lateral semicircular canal in this case.

Pathology

In KO, keratin is shed circumferentially, leading to an onionskin-like lamellar arrangement. The removed plug contains tightly packed squames, i.e., flakes of skin. However,

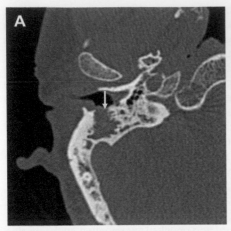 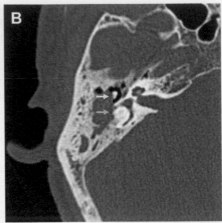

Fig. 4. *Imaging appearance of external auditory canal cholesteatoma.* Noncontrasted computed tomography of the temporal bone (right ear, axial sections). Advanced canal cholesteatoma demonstrating (*A*) erosion of the posterior bony canal wall (yellow *arrow*), and (*B*) erosion into the short process of the incus (yellow *arrow*) and lateral semicircular canal (blue *arrow*), resulting in symptomatic vertigo.

in EACC, keratin sheds from the cholesteatoma sac and is expelled randomly in all directions. On histopathologic analysis, the squames are loosely packed and non-lamellar.[3] Furthermore, in EACC the subepithelial layer demonstrates infiltration with chronic inflammatory cells.[24] If there is diagnostic uncertainty, EACC specimens can be sent for pathologic analysis in order to rule out malignant tumors, such as squamous cell carcinoma of the EAC.[25]

Staging

In addition to the imaging staging system by Shin and colleagues[44] described above, a clinical and histopathologic staging system for EACC was described by Naim and colleagues,[25] as later in discussion.

- Stage I: There is hyperplasia and hyperemia of the canal epithelium.
- Stage II: There is localized inflammation of hyperproliferated epithelium and adjacent periosteitis.
  - Stage IIa: There is an intact epithelial surface.
  - Stage IIb: There is excavation of the defected epithelium and denuded bone.
- Stage III: There is destruction of the bony EAC with sequestrated bone.
- Stage IV: There is spontaneous destruction of adjacent anatomical structures, such as the mastoid, skull base, temporomandibular joint, and facial nerve.

Treatment

Three factors must be considered when deciding on the course of treatment for EACC: the patient's hearing, the extent of disease, and the underlying etiology, whether primary/spontaneous or secondary.[41] For secondary EACC, the underlying cause must also be addressed in addition to disease eradication to prevent recurrence.

Shin and colleagues[44] describe a treatment algorithm that can be correlated to the patient's imaging stage.

- Stage I: Managed with local care or canalplasty.

- Stage II: Managed with canalplasty and tympanoplasty.
- Stage III: Managed with canalplasty, mastoidectomy, and optional tympanoplasty. The bony canal wall may be repaired with bone dust.
- Stage IV: Managed with middle fossa or transzygomatic approach depending on the location of disease.

Treatment can also be based on the Naim and colleagues,[25] clinical and histopathological staging.

- Stages I-IIa: Managed with frequent cleaning and use of eardrops with topical antibiotics particularly if there is a superimposed otitis externa.[47] Mineral oil may help soften cerumen around the cholesteatoma matrix.[28,47] Diluted vinegar rinses may also be a useful adjunct for patient self-management.[47,48]
- Stages IIb-III: Managed with transcanal canalplasty.
- Stage IV: Managed with meatocanalplasty and canal wall down mastoidectomy.

The vast majority of patients can typically be managed with routine debridement and medical management of infections as they arise. The most common indication for surgery is either uncertainty in diagnosis (biopsy) or the inability to completely access the complete depth of the cholesteatoma in the clinic. This could be due to the configuration of bony erosion or due to a narrowed meatus.

Complications

EACC may spread to involve surrounding structures, including the temporomandibular joint,[49] middle ear, mastoid, facial nerve,[50] tegmen, and semicircular canals.[51] Intracranial involvement leading to abscess is also possible but fortunately exceedingly rare.[52]

DISCUSSION

There is considerable overlap in the presentations of KO and EACC. Our understanding of these 2 pathologies has come a long way since the first description by Toynbee in 1850.[2] In the majority of cases for both pathologies, conservative management consisting of aural toilet in the clinic is sufficient to reduce symptoms and prevent progression of disease. If disease is extensive, surgery may be required. Surgery is more likely to be required for EACC than it is for KO. When surgery is required for either EACC or KO, the approaches for both are also not dissimilar. Continued research is required to better understand the underlying pathophysiologic mechanisms to enable prevention, personalized treatment, and mitigation of complications.

CLINICS CARE POINTS

- Keratosis obturans (KO) and external auditory canal cholesteatoma (EACC) are discrete but similar keratinaceous lesions of the external auditory canal (EAC).
- KO leads to circumferential widening of the EAC with acute otalgia. On the other hand, EACC leads to focal bony erosion of the EAC, typically of the floor and/or posterior canal wall. It is associated with chronic, dull otalgia and is more often associated with otorrhea than is KO.
- KO is associated with hearing loss. To the contrary, EACC does not typically cause hearing loss if confined to the canal. However, hearing loss may occur if disease spreads to adjacent areas. Hearing loss may also be secondary to the underlying cause in secondary EACC.
- Osteonecrosis and epithelial loss of EACC are key features that distinguish it from KO. The history and physical examination are important in making the diagnosis. Imaging can help

with the differential diagnosis and to determine the extent of disease for both pathologies. Histopathologic analysis may be helpful if there is uncertainty but is not required in every case.

- Both pathologies often respond well to aural toilet in the clinic. If surgery is required for extensive disease (more often for EACC than for KO), the surgical approaches are similar.

DISCLOSURE

T. Munjal serves as a consultant for Spiral Therapeutics for work unrelated to this article and acknowledges the generous support of the T32DC015209 training grant from the National Institutes of Health, United States/National Institute on Deafness and Other Communication Disorders. No relevant financial disclosures. P.J. Kullar, J. Alyono: No relevant financial disclosures.

REFERENCES

1. Kelly KE, Mohs DC. The external auditory canal: anatomy and physiology. Otolaryngol Clin 1996;29(5):725–39.
2. Toynbee J. Specimens of molluscum contagioscoum developed in the external auditory meatus. Lond Med Gaz 1850;46(11):261–4.
3. Naiberg J, Berger G, Hawke M. The pathologic features of keratosis obturans and cholesteatoma of the external auditory canal. Arch Otolaryngol 1984;110(10):690–3.
4. Piepergerdes JC, Kramer BM, Behnke EE. Keratosis obturans and external auditory canal cholesteatoma. Laryngoscope 1980;90(3):383–91.
5. Aaron K, Cooper TE, Warner L, et al. Ear drops for the removal of ear wax. Cochrane Database Syst Rev 2018;(7).
6. Park SY, Jung YH, Oh J-H. Clinical characteristics of keratosis obturans and external auditory canal cholesteatoma. Otolaryngology-Head Neck Surg (Tokyo) 2015;152(2):326–30.
7. Morrison A. Keratosis obturans. J Laryngol Otol 1956;70(5):317–21.
8. Chong A, Raman R. Keratosis obturans: a disease of the tropics? Indian Journal of Otolaryngology and Head & Neck Surgery 2017;69(3):291–5.
9. Alarouj H, AlObaid F, AlBader AK, et al. A recurrent misdiagnosed and maltreated case of keratosis obturans. Case Reports in Otolaryngology 2019;2019.
10. Kumar V, Soni S, Wadhwa V, et al. An unusual case of keratosis obturans presenting with facial nerve paresis. Otolaryngology Case Reports 2022;22:100400.
11. Black JM, Chaytor RG. Wax keratosis in children's ears. Br Med J 1958; 2(5097):673.
12. Revadi G, Prepageran N, Raman R, et al. Epithelial migration on the external ear canal wall in normal and pathologic ears. Otol Neurotol 2011;32(3):504–7.
13. Corbridge RJ, Michaels L, Wright T. Epithelial migration in keratosis obturans. Am J Otolaryngol 1996;17(6):411–4.
14. Lesser T, Gleeson M. Keratosis obturans and primary auditory canal cholesteatoma. Scott-Brown's Otolaryngology Head and Neck Surgery 2008;7:3342–5.
15. Trojanowska A, Drop A, Trojanowski P, et al. External and middle ear diseases: radiological diagnosis based on clinical signs and symptoms. Insights into imaging 2012;3(1):33–48.
16. Shinnabe A, Hara M, Hasegawa M, et al. A comparison of patterns of disease extension in keratosis obturans and external auditory canal cholesteatoma. Otol Neurotol 2013;34(1):91–4.

17. Kuczkowski J, Mikaszewski B, Narożny W. Immunohistochemical and histopathological features of keratosis obturans and cholesteatoma of the external auditory canal. Atypical keratosis obturans. J Laryngol Otol 2004;118(3):249–51.
18. Harounian J, Patel V, Isildak H. Contemporary management of keratosis obturans: a systematic review. J Laryngol Otol 2021;135(9):1–6.
19. Zwemstra M, Ebbens F, de Wolf M, et al. A novel topical treatment for keratosis obturans. Otol Neurotol 2021;42(10):e1503–6.
20. Paparella MM, Goycoolea MV. Canalplasty for chronic intractable external otitis and keratosis obturans. Otolaryngology-Head Neck Surg (Tokyo) 1981;89(3):440.
21. Poudyal P, Nepal G, Yadav SK, et al. Keratosis obturans: a rare cause of facial nerve palsy. Clinical Case Reports 2022;10(2):e05410.
22. Saunders NC, Malhotra R, Biggs N, et al. Complications of keratosis obturans. J Laryngol Otol 2006;120(9):740–4.
23. Rutkowska J, Özgirgin N, Olszewska E. Cholesteatoma definition and classification: a literature review. The journal of international advanced otology 2017;13(2):266.
24. Anthony PF, Anthony WP. Surgical treatment of external auditory canal cholesteatoma. Laryngoscope 1982;92(1):70–5.
25. Naim R, Linthicum F Jr, Shen T, et al. Classification of the external auditory canal cholesteatoma. Laryngoscope 2005;115(3):455–60.
26. Persaud R, Hajioff D, Thevasagayam M, et al. Keratosis obturans and external ear canal cholesteatoma: how and why we should distinguish between these conditions. Clinical Otolaryngology & Allied Sciences 2004;29(6):577–81.
27. Tos M. Manual of middle ear surgery: surgery of the external auditory canal, 3. New York, NY: Thieme Medical Publishers; 1997.
28. Holt JJ. Ear canal cholesteatoma. Laryngoscope 1992;102(6):608–13.
29. Vrabec JT, Chaljub G. External canal cholesteatoma. Otol Neurotol 2000;21(5):608–14.
30. Bonding P, Ravn T. Primary cholesteatoma of the external auditory canal: is the epithelial migration defective? Otol Neurotol 2008;29(3):334–8.
31. He G, Xu Y, Zhu Z. Clinical analysis of pediatric primary external auditory canal cholesteatoma. Int J Pediatr Otorhinolaryngol 2019;118:25–30.
32. Kim CW, Baek S-H, Lee S-H, et al. Clinical characteristics of spontaneous cholesteatoma of the external auditory canal in children comparing with cholesteatoma in adults. Eur Arch Oto-Rhino-Laryngol 2014;271:3179–85.
33. Casale G, Nicholas BD, Kesser BW. Acquired ear canal cholesteatoma in congenital aural atresia/stenosis. Otol Neurotol 2014;35(8):1474–9.
34. Van Abel KM, Nelson ME, Collar RM, et al. Development of canal cholesteatoma in a patient with prenatal isotretinoin exposure. Int J Pediatr Otorhinolaryngol 2010;74(9):1082–4.
35. Brookes GB, Graham MD. Post-traumatic cholesteatoma of the external auditory canal. Laryngoscope 1984;94(5):667–70.
36. Martin DW, Selesnick SH, Parisier SC. External auditory canal cholesteatoma with erosion into the mastoid. Otolaryngology-Head Neck Surg (Tokyo) 1999;121(3):298–300.
37. Adler M, Hawke M, Berger G, et al. Radiation effects on the external auditory canal. J Otolaryngol 1985;14(4):226–32.
38. Makino K, Amatsu M. Epithelial migration on the tympanic membrane and external canal. Arch Oto-Rhino-Laryngol 1986;243:39–42.
39. Park K, Chun Y-M, Park H-J, et al. Immunohistochemical study of cell proliferation using BrdU labelling on tympanic membrane, external auditory canal and

induced cholesteatoma in mongolian gerbils. Acta Otolaryngol 1999;119(8): 874–9.

40. Yoon YH, Park CH, Eung-Hyub K, et al. Clinical characteristics of external auditory canal cholesteatoma in children. Otolaryngology-Head Neck Surg (Tokyo) 2008;139(5):661–4.

41. Morita S, Nakamaru Y, Fukuda A, et al. Clinical characteristics and treatment outcomes for patients with external auditory canal cholesteatoma. Otol Neurotol 2018;39(2):189–95.

42. Banakis Hartl RM, Said S, Mann SE. Bilateral ear canal cholesteatoma with underlying type I first branchial cleft anomalies. Ann Otol Rhinol Laryngol 2019;128(4): 360–4.

43. Tsuno NS, Tsuno MY, Coelho Neto CA, et al. Imaging the external ear: practical approach to normal and pathologic conditions. Radiographics 2022;42(2): 522–40.

44. Shin S-H, Shim JH, Lee H-K. Classification of external auditory canal cholesteatoma by computed tomography. Clinical and Experimental Otorhinolaryngology 2010;3(1):24–6.

45. van der Meer WL, Waterval JJ, Kunst HP, et al. Diagnosing necrotizing external otitis on CT and MRI: assessment of pattern of extension. Eur Arch Oto-Rhino-Laryngol 2021;279(3):1–6.

46. Mendelson D, Som P, Mendelson M, et al. Malignant external otitis: the role of computed tomography and radionuclides in evaluation. Radiology 1983;149(3): 745–9.

47. Song Y, Jung DH. Office-based management of cholesteatoma. Operat Tech Otolaryngol Head Neck Surg 2021;32(2):127–9.

48. Chang J, Choi J, Im GJ, et al. Dilute vinegar therapy for the management of spontaneous external auditory canal cholesteatoma. Eur Arch Oto-Rhino-Laryngol 2012;269(2):481–5.

49. Salimi F, Motter D, Salimi Z. Temporomandibular joint (TMJ) disorders as first clinical manifestations in external auditory canal cholesteatoma. A case report. Annals of Medicine and Surgery 2022;74:103287.

50. Belcadhi M, Chahed H, Mani R, et al. Therapeutic approaches to complicated cholesteatoma of the external auditory canal: a case of associated facial paresis. Ear Nose Throat J 2010;89(8):E1–6.

51. McCoul ED, Hanson MB. External auditory canal cholesteatoma and keratosis obturans: the role of imaging in preventing facial nerve injury. Ear Nose Throat J 2011;90(12):E1–7.

52. Bhagat S, Varshney S, Bist SS, et al. Primary external auditory canal cholesteatoma presenting as cerebellar abscess. Indian J Otol 2013;19(2):88.

Fungal Infections of the External Auditory Canal and Emerging Pathogens

Erika McCarty Walsh, MD[a],*, Matthew B. Hanson, MD[b]

KEYWORDS

- Otomycosis • Fungal otitis externa • Necrotizing otitis externa
- Malignant otitis externa

KEY POINTS

- Otomycosis is a common fungal infection of the ear canal, and differentiation from bacterial otitis externa is necessary for appropriate treatment.
- Fungal necrotizing otitis externa is of increasing concern in immunocompromised patients, and a high index of suspicion is often required for diagnosis.
- Emerging fungal pathogens of the ear canal are a major public health concern.

BACKGROUND

Fungi are organisms that, with plants, protozoa, chromista and animals, are 1 of the 5 kingdoms of eukaryotes. Fungi are, for the most part, commensal organisms in the human ear, coexisting with us in a symbiotic relationship. In most cases, fungi are saprotrophs, obtaining nutrition by digesting waste produced in the ear canal, most notably the desquamated keratin of our skin cells and the secretions of our sebaceous and ceruminous glands. In rare cases, certain fungi can become pathogens and cause symptoms in the ear canal.

Fungal otitis externa (otomycosis) is the most common fungal disease of the ear canal. Otomycosis may be acute, subacute, or chronic. Fungal disease may account for up to 10% of presentations of otitis externa.[1] Otomycosis is classically described as presenting with pruritus, discharge, and fruiting bodies seen on otomicroscopy, but these symptoms are not universally present. Often, when fungi are seen on microscopy, they are present due to the drainage of pus and mucus from a middle ear infection and are merely growing on this abundant food source and not contributing to the

[a] Department of Otolaryngology, Head and Neck Surgery, University of Alabama at Birmingham, Birmingham, AL, USA; [b] Department of Otolaryngology, SUNY Downstate Health Sciences University, Brooklyn, NY, USA
* Corresponding author. Faculty Office Tower 1155, 1720 2nd Avenue South, Birmingham, AL 35294-3412.
E-mail address: ewalsh@uabmc.edu

Otolaryngol Clin N Am 56 (2023) 909–918
https://doi.org/10.1016/j.otc.2023.06.010
0030-6665/23/© 2023 Elsevier Inc. All rights reserved.

inflammatory process. In fungal otitis externa, however, the bloom of the fungi has itself induced an inflammatory response and is the cause of the symptoms. Patients may present with inflammation and irritation of the ear canal, with white discharge (**Fig. 1**). Decreased hearing and increased tinnitus from canal occlusion and pain may be prominent features in some patients, especially those with immunosuppression.[2] Symptom overlap with acute bacterial otitis externa can make differentiating the 2 challenging, and fungal otitis externa should be suspected if patients with acute otitis externa fail to respond to ototopical antibiotics. Skin fungi, mostly forms of yeast, will particularly be drawn to a warm, moist environment, especially if it has been cleared of the protective wax that typically coats the ear canal. Tropical and subtropical environments may predispose patients to develop otomycosis, although data are conflicting on a regional predilection.[3,4] Acute fungal otitis externa is more common during warmer months of the year.[4] Fungal pathogens have been implicated in chronic otitis externa, especially in cases of chronic manipulation of the ear canal or use of occlusive ear molds.[5,6] Mastoid cavities in particular may be more likely to develop otomycosis. Ototopical antibiotics, especially fluoroquinolone drops, may predispose patients to develop otomycosis by introducing moisture, increasing the ear canal pH, and altering the normal ear canal flora.[3,7,8] Excess moisture and injury to the healthy epithelial layer of the canal are important factors in the development of otomycosis.

Fungi are generally not invasive, but in certain conditions, they can become serious pathogens. In contrast to otomycosis, fungal necrotizing (malignant) otitis externa is a less common but life-threatening cause of ear canal disease. Fungal necrotizing otitis externa is an invasive fungal osteomyelitis of the skull base. Fungal necrotizing otitis

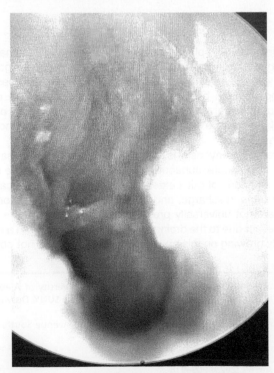

Fig. 1. Otomycosis of the ear on otoendoscopy. Note the absence of fruiting bodies and prominent canal irritation and discharge.

externa may be clinically indistinguishable from bacterial causes of skull base osteo-myelitis, presenting with pain, cranial nerve palsies, granulation tissue at the bony-cartilaginous junction of the ear canal, and intracranial or vascular involvement. Fungal necrotizing otitis externa is often seen in immunocompromised patients, including those with diabetes mellitus, history of organ transplantation, hematologic malig-nancy, and human immunodeficiency virus, and patients who require immunosup-pressive medication.[9] A high index of suspicion is required to identify fungal causes of necrotizing otitis externa.

Clinical Considerations

In cases of otomycosis it is often difficult to identify the pathogen. *Candida* and *Asper-gillus* species have a characteristic and familiar appearance and are the most common fungi identified in otomycosis.[4,10] Candidal infections, in particular, will not present with the dark fruiting bodies in classic description of otomycosis but rather as the typical white, pasty debris overlying erythematous skin as seen elsewhere in the body. *Candida* species infections may be responsible for nearly half of the cases of otomycosis.[10] Fungal pathogens are not usually seen on Gram stains, may be missed by traditional ear canal culture, or may be difficult to differentiate from fungal coloni-zation in chronically moist ears.[11,12] As a result, fungal pathogens may be underrep-resented in studies relying on traditional culture techniques to identify ear canal pathogens. Next-generation DNA sequencing of ears with otitis externa, particularly using polymerase chain reaction sequencing of the large subunit rRNA, suggests that polyfungal infections may occur in as many as 9% of patients.[13] Traditionally, *Aspergillus niger* was reported to be the most common *Aspergillus* species in otomy-cosis, but with improved fungal identification techniques, other species, including *Aspergillus tubingensis*, seem to play a dominant role. Higher rates of resistance to systemic antifungals and higher mean inhibitory concentrations of clotrimazole on susceptibility studies have been reported in *A tubingensis*.[14] In agreement with this, retrospective reviews have suggested that *Aspergillus* infection of the ear canal may be slower to respond to topical antifungals, such as clotrimazole, when compared with candida infection.[15] Improved fungal identification techniques will continue to help guide targeted therapy for otomycosis.

Fungal otitis externa may be an underrecognized cause of tympanic membrane perforation. In patients with otomycosis, ear canal debris, patient discomfort, and ca-nal edema may limit examination of the tympanic membrane. Direct inoculation of the tympanic membrane by fungal pathogens in the ear canal is thought to lead to mycotic thrombus and ischemia and necrosis of the tympanic membrane.[16] The incidence of tympanic membrane perforation in patients with otomycosis may exceed 10%.[17] Immunosuppressed patients in particular may be more likely to develop a tympanic membrane perforation in the setting of otomycosis.[18] Otomycosis should be treated before any attempt at myringoplasty or tympanoplasty, and potential ototoxicity of any topical treatment should be considered carefully in patients with otomycosis.[17] However, with good control of fungal otitis externa, most perforations secondary to otomycosis will heal without intervention.[16,19]

Ear canal debridement, aural toilet, and topical antifungal or antiseptic therapy are the mainstays of treatment of otomycosis. Even though otomycosis is a common diag-nosis seen in the otolaryngology clinic, there are few high-quality randomized controlled trials evaluating the treatment of otomycosis. Clotrimazole is the most com-mon topical antifungal medication used in otomycosis and is available as a solution, cream, and powder with high cure rates reported in multiple studies.[20-30] Clotrimazole preparations are inexpensive and generally widely available. Clotrimazole 1% topical solution is frequently prescribed for home application in patients with otomycosis, but it may burn, limiting patient adherence to treatment.[23] After debridement under otomicroscopic guidance, a single application of topical azole cream or ointment with a syringe and angiocathether can be a simple form of treatment requiring less patient effort and adherence (**Fig. 2**). Patients can return to clinic within 3 to 7 days to remove the excess. A single application of 1% clotrimazole has been reported to result in short-term resolution of otomycosis in up to 95% of patients.[20,22] Despite small retrospective and prospective studies demonstrating benefit to topical antifungal therapy, a recent Cochrane systematic review concluded there was insufficient evidence to conclude that topical azoles are superior to no treatment or that clotrimazole is superior to other, less-available topical azoles.[31] Oral antifungals, such as voriconazole, have rarely been used in refractory cases of otomycosis but come with concerns about systemic side effects and toxicity.[32] Topical acidification and antiseptic agents, including boric acid, povidone-iodine, acetic acid, and silver nitrate gel have been used in otomycosis, with generally good rates of success.[27,29,30,33–36] Otomycosis is often slower to resolve than acute bacterial otitis externa, and repeat visits for debridement are often required.[37] Careful counseling of patients about the need for repeat debridement, aural toilet, avoidance of moisture and ear canal manipulation, and potential need for repeat topical therapy can help patients set appropriate expectations and improve treatment adherence.

Classically, *Pseudomonas aeruginosa* is the most commonly cited pathogen in cases of necrotizing or malignant otitis externa.[38] However, fungal causes of necrotizing externa may be more important than previously thought. Upward of a third of necrotizing otitis externa may be due to fungal pathogens, and fungal causes of necrotizing otitis externa may be on the rise, although the reason for this remains unclear.[39,40] *Aspergillus* species and *Candida albicans* are most commonly identified in fungal necrotizing otitis externa.[41] Fungal pathogens may be missed in necrotizing fungal otitis externa and skull base osteomyelitis, with 60% of invasive *Aspergillus* infections missed by traditional fungal culture.[9] In a series of 19 patients, those with culture-negative necrotizing otitis externa were tested with polymerase chain reaction assays, and all culture-negative patients were found to have evidence of fungal infection missed by traditional culture techniques.[42] Fungal necrotizing otitis externa may

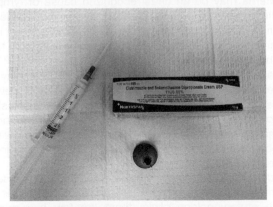

Fig. 2. Setup for in-office application of topical clotrimazole/betamethasone for otomycosis. A 3-mL syringe is filled with the topical cream and fitted with a 16-gauge angiocatheter. Under otomicroscopic guidance, after debridement, the entire ear canal is completely filled with the topical preparation. The patient is instructed to keep the ear dry and may return in several days for removal of residual cream.

only be recognized once treatment directed at bacterial pathogens fails.[43] Patients with fungal necrotizing otitis externa may be particularly resistant to treatment, even when the correct pathogen is identified.[44] Patients may also have a more aggressive disease course, with higher rates of facial palsy, younger age at presentation, higher rate of disease relapse despite appropriate antifungal therapy, and lower 5-year survival than patients with bacterial disease.[45,46] In contrast to otomycosis, fungal necrotizing otitis externa often requires both surgical debridement and systemic antifungal treatment.[44] Surgical intervention may provide the opportunity to not only debride necrotic tissue but also obtain tissue for culture to ensure identification of fungal pathogens, although this remains controversial.[43,47]

Emerging fungal infections of the ear canal deserve mention. *Candida auris* is a multidrug-resistant yeast first identified in 2009 from the draining ear of a hospitalized patient in Japan.[48] *C auris* has now been reported worldwide, especially in hospital settings, and is an emerging nosocomial pathogen of particular concern.[49,50] Patients may present with otorrhea or chronic otitis externa, and fungemia is a frequent complication. High rates of resistance to traditional systemic antifungals, even to potent antifungals such as amphotericin B, have been reported. *C auris* is difficult to identify in the microbiology laboratory, and mortality rates of invasive infection exceed 50%.[51]

Individual patient factors may play a role in the development of both otomycosis and fungal necrotizing otitis externa. Next-generation DNA sequencing comparing normal and diseased ears suggests fundamental changes to the mycobiome of the ear in patients with otitis externa.[13] Patients with *Aspergillus* osteomyelitis of the skull base were found to have decreased production of interleukin (IL)-17 and IL-22, cytokines integral to the Th17 helper T-cell response to fungal pathogens.[52] There may be other host factors yet to be identified that predispose patients to fungal infections of the ear canal. Further research is needed to understand more precisely which patients are most vulnerable to fungal infections of the ear canal.

Fungi have also been found to be a factor in several disorders previously thought to be dermatologic in nature. *Malassezia* is yeast that is ubiquitous and is a frequent resident of human sebaceous glands.[53] This organism is incapable of making large-chain lipids and is therefore dependent on a plentiful source of lipid for survival. This feature makes it difficult to culture, and its role in several dermatologic conditions was not known until recently. Atopic dermatitis, seborrheic dermatitis, folliculitis, and pityriasis versicolor are all now attributed to *Malassezia*. It is unknown what turns this normally commensal organism into a pathogen, but it is thought to be related to an interaction with the immune system.

Another pathologic condition unique to fungi is the so-called id reaction; this is an eczematous reaction to a fungal infection elsewhere in the body.[54] This reaction is most frequent with dermatophyte infections such as ringworm or athlete's foot but can also be seen in candida infections. This pathologic condition will present as an eczematous lesion, but it will not be responsive to steroid therapy. The lesion resolves when the primary infection is treated. Cases of an id reaction as a cause of ear canal dermatitis have been reported in the ENT literature.[55]

DISCUSSION

Providers should be on high alert for fungal infections of the ear canal. Otomycosis, the most common fungal infection of the ear canal, can mimic bacterial otitis externa and chronic otitis externa, and fungal necrotizing otitis externa can be clinically indistinguishable from bacterial infections. Fungal necrotizing otitis externa may be even more common than previously realized, and failure to identify a fungal cause can have a devastating effect on patient outcomes.[44–46] Although it is tempting to try to use basic culture techniques to differentiate fungal and bacteria pathogens, data suggest that traditional culture techniques often fail to identify fungal infections of the ear canal.[9,11,12,42] Tissue biopsy and culture should be considered, especially in cases of necrotizing otitis externa. Providers should be particularly suspicious for fungal infections in patients who fail to respond to therapy, have atypical presentations, or have known risk factors for fungal infections.

There are several known or suspected patient factors that can predispose patients to fungal infections of the ear canal. Diabetes, history of transplant, hematologic malignancy, and use of immunosuppressant medications are all risk factors for local but especially invasive fungal disease.[9] Patients in hospital or institutional settings are more likely to develop *C. auris* infection. However, more investigation is needed to fully understand whether patient differences in immune response or other inherent factors place patients at particular risk of fungal infections of the ear canal.

SUMMARY

Otomycosis is a common fungal infection of the ear canal, and differentiation from bacterial otitis externa is necessary for appropriate treatment. Aural toilet, ear canal debridement, and ototopical antifungals are accepted forms of treatment of otomycosis. Fungal necrotizing otitis externa is of increasing concern in immunocompromised patients, and a high index of suspicion is often required for diagnosis. Emerging fungal pathogens of the ear canal are a major public health concern. Further studies are needed to guide best practices in fungal ear canal infections.

CLINICS CARE POINTS

- Otomycosis may not always present with classic symptoms of pruritus and visible fungal fruiting bodies
- Otomycosis is treated with a combination of mechanical debridement and appropriate topical therapy
- Single application of 1% clotrimazole cream or similar in otomycosis may be curative in many patients and does not require strict patient adherence
- Fungal necrotizing otitis externa may be more common than previously appreciated and may have worse clinical outcomes
- Fungal pathogens may be missed by traditional culture techniques, and tissue culture may be required in severe disease
- *C. auris* is an emerging, drug-resistant fungal cause of otitis externa often found in health care settings

DISCLOSURE

The author has no relevant disclosures.

REFERENCES

1. Ho T, Vrabec JT, Yoo D, et al. Otomycosis: clinical features and treatment implications. Otolaryngol Head Neck Surg 2006;135(5):787–91. https://doi.org/10.1016/j.otohns.2006.07.008.

2. Viswanatha B, Sumatha D, Vijayashree MS. Otomycosis in immunocompetent and immunocompromised patients: comparative study and literature review. Ear Nose Throat J 2012;91(3):114–21. https://doi.org/10.1177/014556131209100308.

3. Munguia R, Daniel SJ. Ototopical antifungals and otomycosis: a review. Int J Pediatr Otorhinolaryngol 2008;72(4):453–9. https://doi.org/10.1016/j.ijporl.2007.12.005.

4. Roland PS, Stroman DW. Microbiology of acute otitis externa. Laryngoscope 2002;112(7 Pt 1):1166–77. https://doi.org/10.1097/00005537-200207000-00005.

5. Hawke M, Wong J, Krajden S. Clinical and microbiological features of otitis externa. J Otolaryngol 1984;13(5):289–95.

6. Orji FT, O Onyero E, Agbo CE. The clinical implications of ear canal debris in hearing aid users. Pak J Med Sci 2014;30(3):483–7. https://doi.org/10.12669/pjms.303.4742.

7. Alshahni MM, Alshahni RZ, Fujisaki R, et al. A Case of Topical Ofloxacin-Induced Otomycosis and Literature Review. Mycopathologia 2021;186(6):871–6. https://doi.org/10.1007/s11046-021-00581-x.

8. Jackman A, Ward R, April M, et al. Topical antibiotic induced otomycosis. Int J Pediatr Otorhinolaryngol 2005;69(6):857–60. https://doi.org/10.1016/j.ijporl.2005.01.022.

9. Macias D, Jeong SS, Van Swol JM, et al. Trends and Outcomes of Fungal Temporal Bone Osteomyelitis: A Scoping Review. Otol Neurotol 2022;43(10):1095–107. https://doi.org/10.1097/MAO.0000000000003714.

10. Pontes ZBV da S, Silva ADF, Lima E de O, et al. Otomycosis: a retrospective study. Braz J Otorhinolaryngol 2009;75(3):367–70. https://doi.org/10.1016/S1808-8694(15)30653-4.

11. Saunders JE, Raju RP, Boone JL, et al. Antibiotic resistance and otomycosis in the draining ear: culture results by diagnosis. Am J Otolaryngol 2011;32(6):470–6. https://doi.org/10.1016/j.amjoto.2010.09.009.

12. Rawson TM, Fatania N, Abdolrasouli A. UK standards for microbiology investigations of ear infection (SMI B1) are inadequate for the recovery of fungal pathogens and laboratory diagnosis of otomycosis: A real-life prospective evaluation. Mycoses 2022;65(4):490–5. https://doi.org/10.1111/myc.13423.

13. Burton M, Krumbeck JA, Wu G, et al. The adult microbiome of healthy and otitis patients: Definition of the core healthy and diseased ear microbiomes. PLoS One 2022;17(1):e0262806. https://doi.org/10.1371/journal.pone.0262806.

14. Kamali Sarvestani H, Seifi A, Falahatinejad M, et al. Black aspergilli as causes of otomycosis in the era of molecular diagnostics, a mini-review. J Mycol Med 2022;32(2):101240. https://doi.org/10.1016/j.mycmed.2021.101240.

15. Antunes J, Mendes N, Adónis C, et al. Treatment of otomycosis with clotrimazole: results accordingly with the fungus isolated. Acta Otolaryngol 2022;142(9–12):664–7. https://doi.org/10.1080/00016489.2022.2117845.

16. Hurst WB. Outcome of 22 cases of perforated tympanic membrane caused by otomycosis. J Laryngol Otol 2001;115(11):879–80. https://doi.org/10.1258/0022215011909486.

17. Koltsidopoulos P, Skoulakis C. Otomycosis With Tympanic Membrane Perforation: A Review of the Literature. Ear Nose Throat J 2020;99(8):518–21. https://doi.org/10.1177/0145561319851499.

18. Rutt AL, Sataloff RT. Aspergillus otomycosis in an immunocompromised patient. Ear Nose Throat J 2008;87(11):622–3.

19. Song JE, Haberkamp TJ, Patel R, et al. Fungal otitis externa as a cause of tympanic membrane perforation: a case series. Ear Nose Throat J 2014;93(8):332–6. https://doi.org/10.1177/014556131409300811.

20. Chavan RP, Ingole SM, Kanchewad Resident GS. Single Topical Application of 1% Clotrimazole Cream in Otomycosis. Indian J Otolaryngol Head Neck Surg 2022;1–8. https://doi.org/10.1007/s12070-022-03206-x.

21. de la Paz Cota BR, Cepero Vega PP, Matus Navarrete JJ, et al. Efficacy and safety of eberconazole 1% otic solution compared to clotrimazole 1% solution in patients with otomycosis. Am J Otolaryngol 2018;39(3):307–12. https://doi.org/10.1016/j.amjoto.2018.03.017.

22. Dundar R, İynen İ. Single Dose Topical Application of Clotrimazole for the Treatment of Otomycosis: Is This Enough? J Audiol Otol 2019;23(1):15–9. https://doi.org/10.7874/jao.2018.00276.

23. Haq M, Deshmukh P. Review of Recurrent Otomycosis and Clotrimazole in Its Treatment. Cureus 2022;14(10):e30098. https://doi.org/10.7759/cureus.30098.

24. Herasym K, Bonaparte JP, Kilty S. A comparison of Locacorten-Vioform and clotrimazole in otomycosis: A systematic review and one-way meta-analysis. Laryngoscope 2016;126(6):1411–9. https://doi.org/10.1002/lary.25761.

25. Jimenez-Garcia L, Celis-Aguilar E, Díaz-Pavón G, et al. Efficacy of topical clotrimazole vs. topical tolnaftate in the treatment of otomycosis. A randomized controlled clinical trial. Braz J Otorhinolaryngol 2020;86(3):300–7. https://doi.org/10.1016/j.bjorl.2018.12.007.

26. Kiakojuri K, Mahdavi Omran S, Roodgari S, et al. Molecular Identification and Antifungal Susceptibility of Yeasts and Molds Isolated from Patients with Otomycosis. Mycopathologia 2021;186(2):245–57. https://doi.org/10.1007/s11046-021-00537-1.

27. Mofatteh MR, Naseripour Yazdi Z, Yousefi M, et al. Comparison of the recovery rate of otomycosis using betadine and clotrimazole topical treatment. Braz J Otorhinolaryngol 2018;84(4):404–9. https://doi.org/10.1016/j.bjorl.2017.04.004.

28. Nemati S, Gerami H, Faghih Habibi A, et al. Sertaconazole versus Clotrimazole and Miconazole Creams in the Treatment of Otomycosis: A Placebo-Controlled Clinical Trial. Iran J Otorhinolaryngol 2022;34(120):27–34. https://doi.org/10.22038/IJORL.2021.54805.2872.

29. Philip A, Thomas R, Job A, et al. Effectiveness of 7.5 percent povidone iodine in comparison to 1 percent clotrimazole with lignocaine in the treatment of otomycosis. ISRN Otolaryngol 2013;2013:239730. https://doi.org/10.1155/2013/239730.

30. Romsaithong S, Tomanakan K, Tangsawad W, et al. Effectiveness of 3 per cent boric acid in 70 per cent alcohol versus 1 per cent clotrimazole solution in otomycosis patients: a randomised, controlled trial. J Laryngol Otol 2016;130(9):811–5. https://doi.org/10.1017/S0022215116008598.

31. Lee A, Tysome JR, Saeed SR. Topical azole treatments for otomycosis. Cochrane Database Syst Rev 2021;5(5):CD009289. https://doi.org/10.1002/14651858.CD009289.pub2.

32. Ho HC, Hsiao SH, Lee CY, et al. Treatment of refractory Aspergillus otomycosis with voriconazole: case series and review. J Laryngol Otol 2014;128(6):547–51. https://doi.org/10.1017/S0022215114001273.

33. del Palacio A, Cuétara MS, López-Suso MJ, et al. Randomized prospective comparative study: short-term treatment with ciclopiroxolamine (cream and solution) versus boric acid in the treatment of otomycosis. Mycoses 2002;45(8):317–28. https://doi.org/10.1046/j.1439-0507.2002.00737.x.

34. Swain SK, Behera IC, Sahu MC, et al. Povidone iodine soaked gelfoam for the treatment of recalcitrant otomycosis - Our experiences at a tertiary care teaching hospital of eastern India. J Mycol Med 2018;28(1):122–7. https://doi.org/10.1016/j.mycmed.2017.11.006.
35. Wu S, Cheng Y, Lin S, et al. A Comparison of Antifungal Drugs and Traditional Antiseptic Medication for Otomycosis Treatment: A Systematic Review and Meta-Analysis. Front Surg 2021;8:739360. https://doi.org/10.3389/fsurg.2021.739360.
36. Xu H, Liang F ya, Chen L, et al. Evaluation of the utricular and saccular function using oVEMPs and cVEMPs in BPPV patients. J Otolaryngol Head Neck Surg 2016;45:12. https://doi.org/10.1186/s40463-016-0125-7.
37. Martin TJ, Kerschner JE, Flanary VA. Fungal causes of otitis externa and tympanostomy tube otorrhea. Int J Pediatr Otorhinolaryngol 2005;69(11):1503–8. https://doi.org/10.1016/j.ijporl.2005.04.012.
38. Byun YJ, Patel J, Nguyen SA, et al. Necrotizing Otitis Externa: A Systematic Review and Analysis of Changing Trends. Otol Neurotol 2020;41(8):1004–11. https://doi.org/10.1097/MAO.0000000000002723.
39. Glikson E, Sagiv D, Wolf M, et al. Necrotizing otitis externa: diagnosis, treatment, and outcome in a case series. Diagn Microbiol Infect Dis 2017;87(1):74–8. https://doi.org/10.1016/j.diagmicrobio.2016.10.017.
40. Peled C, El-Seid S, Bahat-Dinur A, et al. Necrotizing Otitis Externa-Analysis of 83 Cases: Clinical Findings and Course of Disease. Otol Neurotol 2019;40(1):56–62. https://doi.org/10.1097/MAO.0000000000001986.
41. Di Lullo AM, Russo C, Grimaldi G, et al. Skull Base Fungal Osteomyelitis: A Case Report and Review of the Literature. Ear Nose Throat J 2021;100(10_suppl):1089S–94S. https://doi.org/10.1177/0145561320936006.
42. Gruber M, Roitman A, Doweck I, et al. Clinical utility of a polymerase chain reaction assay in culture-negative necrotizing otitis externa. Otol Neurotol 2015;36(4):733–6. https://doi.org/10.1097/MAO.0000000000000563.
43. Carfrae MJ, Kesser BW. Malignant otitis externa. Otolaryngol Clin North Am 2008;41(3):537–49. https://doi.org/10.1016/j.otc.2008.01.004, viii-ix.
44. Margulis I, Cohen-Kerem R, Roitman A, et al. Laboratory and imaging findings of necrotizing otitis externa are associated with pathogen type and disease outcome: A retrospective analysis. Ear Nose Throat J 2022. https://doi.org/10.1177/01455613221080973. 1455613221080973.
45. Danjou W, Chabert P, Perpoint T, et al. Necrotizing external otitis: analysis of relapse risk factors in 66 patients managed during a 12 year period. J Antimicrob Chemother 2022;77(9):2532–5. https://doi.org/10.1093/jac/dkac193.
46. Hamzany Y, Soudry E, Preis M, et al. Fungal malignant external otitis. J Infect 2011;62(3):226–31. https://doi.org/10.1016/j.jinf.2011.01.001.
47. Takata J, Hopkins M, Alexander V, et al. Systematic review of the diagnosis and management of necrotising otitis externa: Highlighting the need for high-quality research. Clin Otolaryngol 2023. https://doi.org/10.1111/coa.14041.
48. Satoh K, Makimura K, Hasumi Y, et al. Candida auris sp. nov., a novel ascomycetous yeast isolated from the external ear canal of an inpatient in a Japanese hospital. Microbiol Immunol 2009;53(1):41–4. https://doi.org/10.1111/j.1348-0421.2008.00083.x.
49. Araúz AB, Caceres DH, Santiago E, et al. Isolation of Candida auris from 9 patients in Central America: Importance of accurate diagnosis and susceptibility testing. Mycoses 2018;61(1):44–7. https://doi.org/10.1111/myc.12709.

50. Schelenz S, Hagen F, Rhodes JL, et al. First hospital outbreak of the globally emerging Candida auris in a European hospital. Antimicrob Resist Infect Control 2016;5:35. https://doi.org/10.1186/s13756-016-0132-5.
51. Jeffery-Smith A, Taori SK, Schelenz S, et al. Candida auris: a Review of the Literature. Clin Microbiol Rev 2018;31(1). https://doi.org/10.1128/CMR.00029-17. 000299-e117.
52. Delsing CE, Becker KL, Simon A, et al. Th17 cytokine deficiency in patients with Aspergillus skull base osteomyelitis. BMC Infect Dis 2015;15:140. https://doi.org/10.1186/s12879-015-0891-2.
53. Ashbee HR. Update on the genus Malassezia. Med Mycol 2007;45:287–303.
54. Ilkit M, Durdu M, Karakas M. Cutaneous id reactions: a comprehensive review of clinical manifestations, epidemiology, etiology and management. Crit Rev Microbiol 2012;(3):191–202.
55. Derenbery K, Berliner KI. Foot and ear disease–the dermatophytid reaction in otology. Laryngoscope 1996;(2 Pt1):181–6.

Acquired Stenosis of the External Ear Canal

Gauri Mankekar, MD, PhD*, Payam Entezami, MD

KEYWORDS

- Acquired stenosis external ear canal • Canalplasty • Meatoplasty • Skin grafts
- Stents

KEY POINTS

- Acquired external ear canal stenosis can result from multiple causes such as infections, inflammation, accidental or iatrogenic trauma, benign or malignant tumors, and radiation therapy.
- Clinically, patients present with recurrent otorrhea, conductive hearing loss, cerumen impaction and even canal cholesteatoma.
- Surgery is the mainstay for treatment.
- Long term outcomes are unpredictable and range from successful recanalization with hearing improvement to restenosis with worsening conductive hearing loss.

INTRODUCTION

Acquired stenosis of the external ear canal (ASEEC) can result from many causes which initiate a cascade of inflammatory tissue reactions resulting in stenosis of the ear canal.[1] Stenosis or narrowing of the external ear canal (EAC) occurs lateral to the tympanic membrane resulting in a skin lined blind canal.[1] It typically presents as recurrent otorrhea, conductive hearing loss, often with significant cerumen impaction and ear canal cholesteatoma. Different etiologies such as chronic otitis externa, dermatologic diseases, iatrogenic (previous ear surgery or radiotherapy) or accidental trauma, tumor and inflammation have been implicated in its causation. ASEEC involve either the outer ear canal (eg. after trauma) or medial ear canal (eg post-inflammation) or both and can cause conductive hearing loss. History, clinical examination, audiometry, and Computed tomography (CT) scan help to confirm the diagnosis, extent of the stenosis and middle ear status. Diffusion weighted magnetic resonance imaging (DWI MRI) may be required to determine the presence and extent of cholesteatoma. Although medical treatment can be attempted, surgery is the primary modality for

Department of Otolaryngology-Head Neck Surgery, Louisiana State University Health, Shreveport, LA, USA
* Corresponding author. 1501, King's Highway, Shreveport, LA.
E-mail address: gauri.mankekar@lsuhs.edu

Otolaryngol Clin N Am 56 (2023) 919–931
https://doi.org/10.1016/j.otc.2023.06.012
0030-6665/23/© 2023 Elsevier Inc. All rights reserved.

treatment. Several techniques excising scar tissue completely or partially, with or without skin grafting and with and without stenting of the ear canal have been described in literature. Recurrence with restenosis is the most common complication. Stable, long-term outcomes can be challenging in some patients.[2] This article reviews the historical background, prevalence, etiopathogenesis, medical and surgical management of this condition and discusses future trends.

HISTORY/BACKGROUND

- The earliest clinical description of postinflammatory ASEEC ("atresia) was published by Novick in 1939.[3]
- John Conley described "atresia" of the external auditory canal in 10 military personnel after gunshot wounds and other traumas in 1946.[4] He classified the stenosis as web type, solid fibrous healed type, solid fibrous and bony healed type and advocated an endaural approach, excision of scar tissue, application of a thin, split, free skin graft and packing the ear canal with rubber foam impregnated with sulfonamide or penicillin compound.[4]
- Proud in 1955, recommended the terminology "stricture" (Latin "stringere" meaning to "draw tight") for acquired ear canal closure, to avoid confusing the nomenclature of congenital ear canal agenesis or aplasia with the acquired abnormality[5] He also reported successful surgical corrections of acquired ear canal stenosis without prosthetic devices, using endaural approach, radical mastoidectomy, wide meatoplasty and split thickness grafts from the thigh to line the cavity.[5]
- In 1960, Gundersen and in 1965, Eichel and Simonton published case reports describing the treatment of ASEEC caused by chronic otitis externa.[6,7]
- In 1966, Paparella suggested removal of all diseased skin, widening the bony canal maximally with a dental bur, excision of skin with conchal cartilage and replacement with split thickness skin graft using microsurgical tympanoplasty techniques.[8] His report provided the first detailed description of the histology of the tissue excised from the stenosed ear canal. He reported that it showed subepidermal infiltrate of chronic inflammatory cells, predominantly histiocytes. A narrow band of condensed fibrous connective tissue separated the epidermis and the inflammatory cells. The overlying epidermis showed cellular edema and the dermal tissues appeared fibrotic and abnormally hyalinized.

PREVALENCE/INCIDENCE

ASEEC (**Fig. 1**) is not a common condition. However, most otolaryngologists encounter it in their practice. In the largest series of patients treated for acquired ear canal stenosis, an incidence of 0.6 cases per 100000 was reported.[9] Most studies report a female preponderance.[2,10–13] Another common finding is the presence of bilateral disease in patients with ASEEC.[10] The average age at presentation is in the fifth decade although 2 cases have been reported in children.[14,15] The incidence of ear canal cholesteatoma in ASEEC varies from 6% to 9%.[2,9,16] Chronic infection was observed to be the leading cause of ASEEC, followed by postsurgical trauma and accidental trauma.[2,16]

NOMENCLATURE

Acquired stenosis of the external ear canal has been described variously by different authors as "EAC atresia"[9,17–19], "medial meatal fibrosis"[20], acquired medial canal

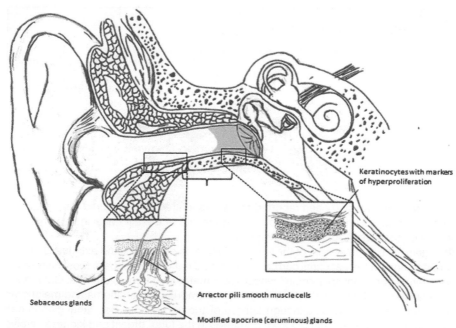

Fig. 1. Acquired stenosis of external ear canal (ASEEC). (*From*: Kmeid M, Nehme J. Post-inflammatory acquired atresia of the external auditory canal. Journal of Otology 2019;14(4): 149 154, see **Fig. 1**.)

fibrosis," "EAC stenosis"[21] and obliterative otitis externa[22,23] representing the different conditions that are caused in this disease process.

ETIOLOGIES AND PATHOGENESIS

In 1943, Conley described 10 cases of posttraumatic ear canal stenosis and classified them into 4 groups: 1. Web type; 2. Solid fibrous healed type; 3. solid fibrous and bony healed type and 4. infected fibrous and bony type.[4]

Tos and Balle classified ASEEC in 1986 and Lavy and colleagues reported it in 2000.[12,15] (**Table 1**). Subsequently various authors sub-classified the condition based on the etiology, as idiopathic, postinflammatory, posttraumatic, iatrogenic (postsurgery or postradiation), neoplastic or dermatologic.[12,20,24–30] (**Table 2**).

Postinflammatory ASEEC accounts for more than 50% of the cases.[2,16] It is a sequelae of chronic otitis media or externa or inflammatory dermatological conditions.[10]

Post-traumatic ASEEC: Accidental blunt trauma such as motor vehicle accidents, penetrating injuries (gunshot wounds) with ear canal lacerations, chemical or thermal burns, fractures involving bony ear canal or posterior displacement of fractures of the head of the mandible can lead to loss of the epidermal lining of the ear canal.[9,12] Circumferential loss of the epidermis heals with granulation tissue formation, followed by fibrosis and subsequent stenosis of the ear canal(**Fig. 2**).[31] Hearing aid molds can cause chronic irritation of the outer ear canal skin, interfere with the normal lateral epithelial migratory pattern of cerumen clearance.[1] The chronic inflammation and lead to chronic otitis externa and eventually lead to stenosis.[32] ASEEC can occur after ear surgery if ear canal skin has been extensively dissected and the periosteum is inadequately covered with the tympanomeatal flap.[33] Overlay myringoplasty with

Table 1
ASEEC classification after Tos et al and Lavy et al[12,15]

1	Post-traumatic atresia	Severe direct trauma, ear contusion, fractures of the anterior wall of the external auditory meatus with the displacement of the mandibular neck
2	Postoperative atresia	Failed meatoplasty postcanal wall down mastoidectomy, severe blunting of the tympanic membrane after myringoplaty
3	Neoplastic atresia	Occlusion of the ear canal by malignant tumor
4	Postinflammatory atresia	Fibrous obliteration of the ear canal following infection, chronic otitis media with otorrhea or external otitis associated with use of hearing aids

lateral blunting has also been reported to be associated with acquired ear canal stenosis.[31,34] Keloids and hypertrophic scars at the site of the ear canal incision are rare causes of *post-ear* surgery canal stenosis.[31,34]

Surgery for benign tumors of the ear canal such as osteomas and exostoses or malignant tumors of the ear canal can cause acquired ear canal stenosis. Most cancers of the external ear canal are primary cancers and metastatic tumors are rare. Cutaneous malignancies such as basal cell carcinoma, squamous cell carcinoma and melanoma are found in the ear canal, although tumors of the ceruminous ear canal glands can also occur.[35] Metastatic tumors from primaries in the lung, breast and kidneys involve the temporal bone due to its vascularity but direct metastasis to the ear canal have also been reported.[35–37]

Surgical treatment of ear canal tumors with circumferential dissection can result in stenosis of the ear canal. Carls and colleagues[30] reported that high dose external beam radiation alone does not predispose patients to external ear canal stenosis. However, there is an increased risk of ear canal stenosis after combined high dose external beam radiation therapy and surgery around the ear canal.[30,38] Other authors have described radiation related osteoradionecrosis of the bony ear canal, sequestration, inflammation of the soft tissue, fibrosis with resulting external otitis and stenosis.[33,39]

Case reports describe external ear canal stenosis resulting from dermatological conditions such as lichen planus, and epidermolysis bullosa affecting the ear canal.[26,29,40] Hopsu and colleagues, postulated an association between auto-immune

Table 2
Modified sub-classification of ASEEC based on etiology[9,15,20]

1	Idiopathic	
2	Postinflammatory	Chronic external otitis due to chronic otorrhea, hearing aid usage
3	Postaccidental trauma	Blunt or penetrating trauma, posterior displaced mandibular head fractures
4	Postiatrogenic trauma	Postear canal surgery for canal wall down mastoidectomy, blunting after overlay myringoplaty, circumferential ear canal surgery for osteoma or exostoses removal, keloids or hypertrophic scars at site of ear canal incisions, radiation of ear canal for parotid, ear canal tumors
5	Neoplastic	Ear canal cutaneous malignancies such as melanoma, basal cell or squamous cell cancers
7	Dermatologic	Lichen Planus, Epidermolysis bullosa

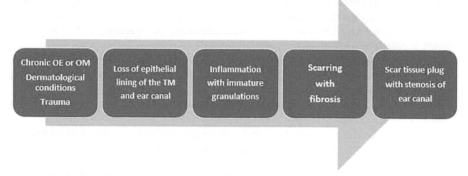

Fig. 2. Pathogenesis of ASEEC -inflammatory cascade.

disorders and medial meatal fibrosis as both lichen planus and ear canal stenosis affect the glabrous skin of the auditory canal and tympanic membrane.[24] Kmeid and colleagues reported acquired ear canal stenosis in two patients with chronic iron deficiency anemia and features of Plummer Vinson syndrome.[41] As the patients responded to systemic iron replacement treatment with improvement in their stenosing external otitis, they suggested a link between iron deficiency anemia and acquired ear canal stenosis.[33]

Most authors *agree that in medial ear canal stenosis* an initial inflammatory process, irrespective of the etiology, triggers loss of the squamous epithelial lining of the medial ear canal. Granular myringitis with the de-epithelialization of the lateral surface of the TM and exposure of the fibrous layer has also been proposed to trigger the inflammatory cascade.[15] Inflammation leads to the production of immature granulation tissue which ultimately matures and forms a firm fibrous plug. The earliest histological description of the tissue was by Paparella.[8] In the absence of inflammation, for example, in post-traumatic cases, the initial trigger is lateral to the tympanic membrane, and heals with the formation of a fibrous, atretic plate, with the entrapment of squamous epithelium and subsequent formation of ear canal cholesteatoma.[42] Bonding and Tos[13] proposed that granulation tissue is formed due to localized inflammation in an isolated area of the ear canal. Epithelialization on either side of the granulation tissue results in membranous atresia and if left untreated, can progress to the formation of a fibrous plug.[13] Kmeid and colleagues have proposed a possible link to iron deficiency anemia and have reported a good response to systemic iron replacement therapy.[33,41]

Lavy and colleagues[15] described 2 stages in the pathogenesis of ASEEC.

- *Primary or Wet stage*: characterized by episodic inflammation, granulations, and recurrent drainage. Organisms such as Pseudomonas and Proteus have been cultured from the drainage. Eventually the granulations heal with fibrosis and stenosis.
- *Secondary or Dry stage* characterized by a thick fibrous plug, with stenosis of external ear canal.

CLINICAL PRESENTATION AND ASSESSMENT

- Hearing loss
- Aural fullness
- Chronic otitis externa

Patients typically present with recurrent otorrhea and progressively worsening hearing loss. There may be discharge with breakdown of the central part.[15] Culture of the discharge shows Pseudomonas and Proteus which are not specific as they are often present in otitis media and chronic otitis media.[14]

A common finding in outer ear canal stenosis is a narrowing of the external meatus, while in medial ear canal stenosis, there may be a solid plug of fibrous tissue occluding view of the tympanic membrane.

Although the condition is typically unilateral, 10-67% of the cases can be bilateral[14,43]

Ear canal cholesteatoma with bone resorption and widening of the floor of the ear canal wall medial to the outer ear canal stenosis has been reported by several authors.[9,17]

Pure tone audiometry shows conductive hearing loss of approximately 30-40dB air bone gap, flat tympanogram and absent stapedial reflexes.[15] Bonding and Tos reported progression of the hearing loss from 15dB to 40dB over 8 years.[13]

IMAGING

High Resolution Computerized tomography (HRCT) scan is most informative for the assessment of the bony ear canal.[44] It helps to evaluate ASEEC, keratosis obturans, cholesteatoma, status of middle ear cavity and ossicles. Typically, the scan will show (**Figs. 3** and **4**) aerated middle ear space, with soft tissue occupying and narrowing the external auditory canal. Traditional and diffusion weighted magnetic resonance imaging is useful to detect concomitant ear canal cholesteatoma.

TREATMENT

Medical management has been supported by Stoney and colleagues,[45] however most of the authors agree that the surgical treatment of ASEEC forms the mainstay of managing the condition.[1,8,12,15]

MEDICAL TREATMENT

Medical management has a limited role, and the goal is to control infection, and prevent progression of granulation tissue to the mature stage. Medical treatment includes aural toilet, topical antibiotic drops, and stenting of the ear canal.

- Although frequent aural toilet is recommended, repeated trauma to the EAC can worsen the condition. Therefore, Luong and colleagues suggested a "no-touch" technique" during aural toilet.[1]

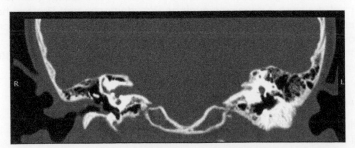

Fig. 3. Coronal CT showing right ear with ASEEC and normal middle ear space.

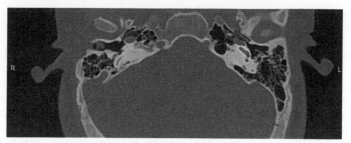

Fig. 4. Axial CT scan showing ASEEC Right ear with cerumen (*white arrow*) plug medial to the stenosis.

- Topical antibiotic drops or powders can be useful to control infection. Luong and colleagues support the use of powders as they adhere to wet surfaces and deliver more stable drug levels.[1]
- Stenting the ear canal with a non-expanding gauze or expanding cellulose wick is typically performed. Miller suggested the use of a soft, expanding cellulose wick to create steady pressure and dilate the ear canal.[46] However, Luong and colleagues observed that a wick has the potential of worsening the inflammatory process due to constant friction with the inflamed EAC.[1]
- Caffior and colleagues proposed using an ear wick with 0.1% tacrolimus ointment every 2nd or 3rd day as an alternative to steroids for the treatment of therapy-resistant otitis externa.[47] They reported clear improvement in 85% of patients short term and complete healing in 46% of their patients at follow-up of 10 -22 months. Magliulo observed that tacrolimus prevented progression of persistent chronic inflammation to mature fibrotic stenosis in his small group of patients with ASEEC.[2]

SURGICAL TREATMENT

Most authors agree that surgical management is necessary to address ASEEC.[8,9,11,15,34,48] Ghani and colleagues recommend surgery in the early wet, granular stage to prevent recurrent ear drainage and disease progression.[49]

Indications for surgery are.

- Failed medical management.
- Progression of the condition to conductive hearing loss

Steps of surgical treatment[15] are.

- Excision of the fibrous plug with the preservation of the fibrous layer of the TM
- Circumferential widening of the ear canal
- Covering the bare bone of the EAC with skin flaps
- Addressing the external ear canal cholesteatoma concomitantly if present.
- Packing of the EAC to maintain patency.

SURGICAL TECHNIQUES

One of the earliest descriptions of surgery for ASEEC was by Conley in 1946. He reported surgical removal of the ear canal plug with recanalization, split thickness skin grafting and sponge packing in 10 young combat soldiers without previous history of ear disease.[4] Paparella and colleagues, in 1966, described postaural approach, canalplasty with circumferential widening of the bony canal using an electric drill followed by a split thickness skin graft.[8] Surgical principles described by Conley[4] and later by Paparella and colleagues[8] have survived the test of time and continue to be used even today, albeit with variations.

Both endaural[31] as well as postaural[31] approaches have been described, although Jacobsen and colleagues[34] reported improved outcomes with the postaural approach. A wedge resection of the fibrous plug was proposed by Soliman and colleagues[50] to prevent postoperative restenosis. However complete excision of the fibrous plug is recommended by most surgeons.[9,13,17,20,43] The fibrous plug is dissected lateral to medially up to the level of the tympanic membrane (TM).[10] The epithelial layer of the TM is denuded, leaving the fibrous layer intact. Generous widening of the bony canal (canalplasty) is performed, meticulously avoiding entering the mastoid air cells or damaging the facial nerve and the temporomandibular joint.[21] Ideally, canalplasty should allow unobstructed view of the tympanomeatal angle and this angle should be at least 90 degrees to prevent scarring.[12] Meatoplasty can be performed at this time to widen the cartilaginous ear canal.

There is consensus about lining the bare ear canal bone, however there is lack of consensus about the best graft to be used. Surgeons have covered the bare ear canal with meatal flaps[51] or regional flaps[51–53] or split (STSG)[34] or full thickness (FTSG)[54] skin grafts. Although FTSG is durable and contains glandular elements,[54] STSGs are preferred by most authors as they are less bulky and have a higher acceptance rate.[4,17,43,55] Some surgeons prefer to harvest the grafts from the arm while others prefer harvesting from the retroauricular area. Depending on the location of the ear canal stenosis, McCary and colleagues[55] used island, segmental or circumferential split thickness skin grafts with excellent long-term results. Adkins and Osguthorpe[52] used transposition flaps in eight cases and reported no recurrences. Retroauricular or preauricular pedicled skin flaps are preferred by some authors.[53,56,57] A well vascularized pedicled flap is associated with a higher rate of graft uptake according to Dhooge and Vermeersch.[58]

Finally, the ear canal is packed to maintain patency. Depending on the surgeon's preference various material have been used for packing and these include gelfoam,[10] or a "Swiss roll" (silastic sheeting with bismuth iodoform soaked ribbon gauze),[34] backing strips, expandable wicks, tracheostomy tube,[59] Foley's catheter,[50] dental impression material,[60] acrylic stents,[61–63] silicon tubes,[19] and drug eluting stents.[64] Matin-Mann et al have proposed a 3D printed, individualized, drug-eluting (dexamethasone, ciprofloxacin, TNF-alpha) external ear canal implant (EECI) to prevent restenosis.[64] Most surgeons remove the packing material after one week, although Soliman and colleagues[50] advocated removal after 6 weeks. The packing material helps to keep the skin graft in place but can completely occlude the external ear canal with resultant hearing loss and can also be a nidus for infections. After removal of the ear canal stent, if the canal appears inflamed, Luong and colleagues recommend placing a Pope wick.[1]

In a retrospective study of 24 patients with ASEEC, Bajin and colleagues[31] reported that the atretic plate was located at the bony-cartilaginous junction in 37.5%, in the cartilaginous canal in 33.3% and rarely in the bony canal. Jacobsen and Mills reported that simple surgical excision of the fibrous plug was inadequate. It was associated with 100% failure in patients studied over a period of 18 years and the use of a split skin graft resulted in a patent ear canal in 70% of the cases.[34]

Battelino and colleagues[65] reported intraoperative application of 1 mL of 0.4 mg/mL of mitomycin C for 4 minutes to the EAC to prevent adhesions and restenosis in a small prospective study. One patient required reapplication postoperatively. Of their 6 ears, 83.3% had adequate patency and improvement in ABG to 10dB or less between 3 and 14 months postop.

CLINICAL OUTCOMES

A successful postoperative outcome is the complete resolution of symptoms with closure of the air-bone gap. In one of the earliest postoperative outcome studies, Becker and Tos compared short- and long-term outcomes. They reported 90% of the patients had an initial air bone gap (ABG) of less than 20dB but this decreased to 61% after two years and 11% of patients had recurrence of ASEEC.[9] The authors also observed that cases with concomitant cholesteatoma had a problematic post-operative course.[9] Irrespective of the surgical technique used, Jacobsen and colleagues[34]'s 18-year follow-up showed recurrence in 21% within one to two years. They observed that 79% of patients had improvement in hearing with decrease in air bone gap from 29 to 17dB on average. However, this hearing improvement decreased over time.[34] In 2009, Magliulo compared his outcomes at twelve months postsurgery and five years postsurgery. He reported that excellent ABG results (ABG 0 to −10dB) decreased from 36% at 6-month follow-up to 12% at 5 years; and failures (ABG >30dB) increased to 24% at 5 years.[2] He concluded that irrespective of the correct surgical procedure, stable, long-term outcomes are unlikely in some patients. Ghani and colleagues[49] reported recurrent otorrhea in 56% of patients, restenosis in 33% and reoccurrence of conductive hearing loss five years after the surgical treatment of ASEEC. Keller and colleagues[10] have proposed 2 reasons for restenosis: 1. Incomplete excision of stenotic fibrous plug or inadequate coverage of denuded bone with skin grafts and 2. Persistent inflammatory disease in the ear canal. Concomitant middle ear disease or conductive deafness secondary to progressive tympanosclerosis after surgical procedure or previous inflammatory disease has been proposed as a cause of the conductive hearing loss in patients with ASEEC.[15] In the absence of a way to predict which patients will develop restenosis or have persistent hearing loss, there is a consensus that patients with ASEEC will require consistent long-term follow-up.[1] Slattery and colleagues[20] reported restenosis 9 years after surgery.

FUTURE DIRECTIONS

ASEEC treatment continues to be challenging. A few reports suggest limited success with topical tacrolimus ointment-soaked wick placement in the ear canal to prevent progression of the disease. Drug eluting stents have been proposed by Matin-Mann et al as proof of concept and may offer hope for ASEEC patients in future. Further research in stents eluting fibroblast activity inhibitors or similar agents in the wet stage of the disease to prevent inflammatory granulations from progressing to fibrosis is needed. Additionally, the development of drug eluting stents for long-term postsurgery use may help to prevent restenosis and worsening of the hearing loss.

SUMMARY

- Chronic otitis externa followed by surgical trauma, tumors, dermatologic conditions, and radiation treatment of head neck cancers can trigger inflammatory cascade leading to ASEEC.
- Complete excision of the stenotic ear canal plug, canaloplasty with or without meatoplasty, re-epithelialization of the EAC with STSGs and stenting of the ear canal are the mainstay of treatment.
- Meticulous postoperative care and prolonged follow-up are necessary.
- Long term clinical outcomes are unpredictable. Restenosis and persistent conductive hearing loss have been reported up to nine years after surgery

CLINICS CARE POINTS

- ASSEEC can involve either bony outer ear canal, medial cartilaginous ear canal or both.
- Aetiology can vary from trauma, tumor to inflammation.
- Clinical examination, Audiometry and CT scan help to diagnose the condition, its extent and degree of hearing loss.
- Surgery forms the mainstay of treatment.

DISCLOSURE

Nothing to disclose.

REFERENCES

1. Luong A, Roland PS. Acquired external auditory canal stenosis: assessment and management. Curr Opin Otolaryngol Head Neck Surg 2005;13(5):273–6.
2. Magliulo G. Acquired atresia of the external auditory canal: recurrence and long-term results. Annals of otology, Rhinology & laryngology 2009;118(5):345–9.
3. Novick JN. Atresia of the external auditory meatus: canalization by electrocoagulation. Arch Otolaryngol 1939;30(5):744–8.
4. Conley JJ. Atresia of the external auditory canal occurring in military service a report on the correction of this condition in ten cases. Arch Otolaryngol 1946; 43:613–22.
5. Proud GO. Stricture of the external auditory canal. Laryngoscope 1956;66:72–84.
6. Eichel BS, Simonton KM. Stenosis of the external auditory meatus secondary to chronic external otitis treated by a simplified surgical method. Laryngoscope 1965;75(1):16–21.
7. Gundersen T. Atresia meatus acusticus externus als folge von otitis externa eczematosa. Acta Otolaryngol 1960;52(1–6):473–6.
8. Paparella MM, Kurkjian JM. Surgical treatment for chronic stenosing external otitis. Laryngoscope 1966;76(2):243–5.
9. Becker BC, Tos M. Postinflammatory acquired atresia of the external auditory canal: treatment and results of surgery over 27 years. Laryngoscope 1998;108(6): 903–7.
10. Keller RG, Ong AA, Nguyen SA, et al. Postinflammatory medial canal fibrosis: an institutional review and meta-analysis of short- and long-term outcomes. Laryngoscope 2017;127(2):488–95.
11. Dhooge I, D'Hoop M, Loose D, et al. Acquired atresia of the external auditory canal: long-term clinical and audiometric results after surgery. Otol Neurotol 2014; 35(7):1196–200.
12. Tos M, Balle V. Postinflammatory acquired atresia of the external auditory canal: late results of surgery. Am J Otol 1986;7(5):365–70.
13. Bonding P, Tos M. Post inflammatory acquired atresia of the external auditory canal. Acta Otolaryngol 1975;79:115–23.
14. Keohane JD, Ruby RR, Janzen VD, et al. Medial meatal fibrosis: the University of Western Ontario experience. Am J Otol 1993;14(2):172–5.
15. Lavy J, Fagan P. Chronic stenosing external otitis/postinflammatory acquired atresia: a review. Clin Otolaryngol Allied Sci 2000;25(6):435–9.

16. Selesnick S, Nguyen TP, Eisenman DJ. Surgical treatment of acquired external auditory canal atresia. Am J Otol 1998;19(2):123–30.
17. Cremers WR, Smeets JH. Acquired atresia of the external auditory canal. Surgical treatment and results. Arch Otolaryngol Head Neck Surg 1993;119(2):162–4.
18. Anthony WP. Congenital and acquired atresia of the external auditory canal. Arch Otolaryngol 1956;65(5):479–86.
19. Beales PH. Atresia of the external auditory meatus. Arch Otolaryngol Head Neck Surg 1974;100(3):209–11.
20. Slattery WH, Saadat P. Post-inflammatory medial canal fibrosis. Am J Otol 1997; 18:294–7.
21. Birman CS, Fagan PA. Medial canal stenosis -chronic stenosing external otitis. Am J Otol 1996;17:2–6.
22. Herdman RCD, Wright JLW. Surgical treatment of obliterative otitis externa. Clin Otolaryngol 1990;15(1):11–4.
23. Potter CPS, Bottrill ID. Outcomes of canalplasty for chronic obliterative otitis externa. J Laryngol Otol 2012;126(10):1016–21.
24. Hopsu E, Pitkäranta A. Idiopathic, inflammatory, medial meatal, fibrotising otitis presenting with lichen planus. J Laryngol Otol 2007;121(8):796–9.
25. Lillie HI, McBean JB. Chronic mastoiditis with cholesteatoma and stenosis of the external auditory meatus; report of two cases. Proc Staff Meet Mayo Clin 1947; 22(12):246–8.
26. Lazzerini F, Bruschini L, Berrettini S, et al. Lichen planus of the external auditory canal: treatment options and review of literature. Clin Case Rep 2020;8(10):2017–20.
27. Sosulski AB, Hayes JD. Cicatricial external auditory canal stenosis caused by ectodermal dysplasia: rapp-hodgkin syndrome. Ear Nose Throat J 2013;92(6):E24–6.
28. Mikals SJ, Huang Z, Reilly BK, et al. Iatrogenic external auditory canal stenosis induced by silver nitrate. Ear Nose Throat J 2018;97(4–5):E39–40.
29. Milani A, Pace A, Iannella G, et al. Recessive dystrophic epidermolysis bullosa: rare bilateral external auditory canal stenosis and surgical treatment. Clin Med Insights Case Rep 2022;15. https://doi.org/10.1177/11795476221131196. 11795476221311.
30. Carls JL, Mendenhall WM, Morris CG, et al. External auditory canal stenosis after radiation therapy. Laryngoscope 2002;112(11):1975–8.
31. Bajin MD, Yilmaz T, Gunaydin RO, et al. Management of acquired atresia of the external auditory canal. J Int Adv Otol 2015;11(2):147–50.
32. Work WP. Lesions of the external auditory canal. AnnOtol Rhin & Laryngol. 1950; 59:1062.
33. Kmeid M, Nehme J. Post-inflammatory acquired atresia of the external auditory canal. J Otol 2019;14(4):149–54.
34. Jacobsen N, Mills R. Management of stenosis and acquired atresia of the external auditory meatus. J Laryngol Otol 2006;120(4):266–71.
35. White RD, Ananthakrishnan G, McKean SA, et al. Masses and disease entities of the external auditory canal: Radiological and clinical correlation. Clin Radiol 2012;67(2):172–81.
36. James A, Karandikar S, Baijal S. External auditory canal lesion: colorectal metastatic adenocarcinoma. BMJ Case Rep 2018. https://doi.org/10.1136/bcr-2018-224876. bcr-2018-224876.
37. Carson HJ, Krivit JS, Eilers SG. Metastasis of colonic adenocarcinoma to the external ear canal: an unusual case with a complex pattern of disease progression. Ear Nose Throat J 2005;84(1):36–8.

38. Carls JL, Mendenhall WM, Morris CG, Antonelli PJ. External auditory canal stenosis after radiation therapy. Laryngoscope 2002;112(11):1975–8.
39. Adler M, Hawke M, Berger G, et al. Radiation effects on the external auditory canal. J Otolaryngol 1985;14(4):226–32.
40. Košec A, Kostić M, Ajduk J, et al. Hypertrophic recurring lichen planus of the external auditory canal. Eur Ann Otorhinolaryngol Head Neck Dis 2019;136(2): 123–6.
41. Kmeid M, Nehme J. Bilateral obliterative external otitis in the context of chronic iron deficiency—report of two cases. Oncology & Hematology Review (US) 2018;14(1):42.
42. Roland PS. Chronic external otitis. Ear Nose Throat J 2001;80(6 Suppl):12–6.
43. McDonald TJ, Facer GW, Clark JL. Surgical treatment of stenosis of the external auditory canal. Laryngoscope 1986;96(8):830–3.
44. Filippkin MA, Kurilenkov GV, Zelikovich EI. [Temporal bone CT in the diagnosis of acquired diseases of the external auditory canal]. Vestn Rentgenol Radiol 2004; 1:10–4.
45. Stoney P, Kwok P, Hawke M. Granular myringitis: a review. J Otolaryngol 1992; 21(2):129–35.
46. Miller GW. Treatment of acute ear canal stenosis with an expanding cellulose wick. Arch Otolaryngol Head Neck Surg 1978;104(1):55–6.
47. Caffier PP, Harth W, Mayelzadeh B, et al. Tacrolimus: a new option in therapy-resistant chronic external otitis. Laryngoscope 2007;117(6):1046–52.
48. Fisch U, Chang P, Linder T. Meatoplasty for lateral stenosis of the external auditory canal. Laryngoscope 2002;112(7):1310–4.
49. Ghani A, Smith MCF. Postinflammatory medial meatal fibrosis: early and late surgical outcomes. J Laryngol Otol 2013;127(12):1160–8.
50. Soliman T, Fatt-Hi A, Kadir MA. A simplified technique for the management of acquired stenosis of the external auditory canal. J Laryngol Otol 1980;94(5):549–52.
51. Wolfensberger M, Hilger PA, Hilger JA. Conchal bowl and postauricular flaps for reconstruction of the external auditory canal. Otolaryngology-Head Neck Surg (Tokyo) 1983;91(4):404–6.
52. Adkins WY, Osguthorpe JD. Management of canal stenosis with a transposition flap. Laryngoscope 1981;91(8):1267–9.
53. Stucker FJ, Shaw GY. Revision meatoplasty: management emphasizing de-epithelialized postauricular flaps. Otolaryngology-Head Neck Surg (Tokyo) 1991; 105(3):433–9.
54. Moore GF, Moore IJ, Yonkers AJ, et al. Use of full thickness skin grafts in canalplasty. Laryngoscope 1984;94(8):1117–8.
55. McCary WS, Kryzer TC, Lambert PR. Application of split-thickness skin grafts for acquired diseases of the external auditory canal. Am J Otol 1995;16(6):801–5.
56. Nagaoka M, Noguchi Y, Kawashima Y, et al. Long-term result of meatoplasty using inferiorly based retroauricular island pedicle flap for external auditory canal stenosis. Auris Nasus Larynx 2016;43(4):382–6.
57. Bell DR. External auditory canal stenosis and atresia: dual flap surgery. J Otolaryngol 1988;17(1):19–21.
58. Dhooge IJM, Vermeersch HFE. The use of two pedicled skin flaps in the surgical treatment of acquired atresia of the outer ear canal 1. Clin Otolaryngol Allied Sci 1999;24(1):58–60.
59. Sian Ng CS, Kin Foong SK, Ping Loong SP, et al. A novel use of modified tracheostomy tubes in preventing external auditory canal stenosis. J Int Adv Otol 2021; 17(4):301–5.

60. Bast F, Chadha P, Shelly J, et al. Prevention of postoperative ear canal stenosis using stents made of dental impression material: a rapid, cost-effective solution. Clin Otolaryngol 2017;42(4):954–6.
61. Savion I, Good J, Sharon-Buller A. An acrylic resin conformer for the prevention of external auditory meatus stenosis. Laryngoscope 2005;115(11):2006–9.
62. Sela M, Feinmesser R, Capany B, et al. Prosthetic repair of meatal stenosis. J Prosthet Dent 1986;56(2):214–6.
63. Hocwald E, Sichel JY, Sela M, et al. Prevention of post-mastoidectomy meatal stenosis by an acrylic prosthesis. Laryngoscope 2002;112(10):1892–4.
64. Matin-Mann F, Gao Z, Schwieger J, et al. Individualized, additively manufactured drug-releasing external ear canal implant for prevention of postoperative restenosis: development, in vitro testing, and proof of concept in an individual curative trial. Pharmaceutics 2022;14(6):1242.
65. Battelino S, Hocevar-Boltezar I, Zargi M. Intraoperative use of mitomycin C in fibrous atresia of the external auditory canal. Ear Nose Throat J 2005;84(12): 776–9.

Congenital Anomalies of the Ear Canal

Daniel Morrison, MD, Bradley Kesser, MD*

KEYWORDS

- Congenital aural atresia • Congenital aural stenosis • Ear canal stenosis
- Aural atresia • Atresiaplasty • Canalplasty • Conductive hearing loss
- First branchial cleft cyst

KEY POINTS

- Congenital aural atresia (CAA) is usually accompanied by microtia and an associated conductive hearing loss.
- Congenital aural stenosis (CAS) is identified on physical exam; evaluation should include audiometry and an assessment of the self-cleaning ability of the canal.
- High-resolution temporal bone computed tomography (CT) imaging is the radiographic study of choice for the surgical evaluation of CAA and CAS.
- First branchial cleft cysts and sinuses present with preauricular swelling and occasional drainage; a high index of suspicion is necessary for the diagnosis.
- There are many options – both surgical and nonsurgical – for hearing habilitation in patients with CAA.

INTRODUCTION

Congenital anomalies of the external auditory canal (EAC) are classically divided into congenital aural atresia (CAA) and congenital aural stenosis (CAS). Type I branchial cleft cysts, sinuses, and fistulae could also be included among congenital anomalies of the ear canal. CAA is an intrauterine developmental anomaly characterized by the complete absence of the EAC or, less commonly, by various degrees of ear canal stenosis. CAA is almost always associated with some degree of deformity of the auricle (microtia; **Fig. 1**) or anotia (absence of the auricle) and maldevelopment of the middle ear and ossicles. CAA is rarely associated with inner ear abnormalities due to the separate embryologic origins of the inner ear (otic placode) from the ear canal and middle ear (branchial apparatus). Furthermore, the implication of these disparate embryologic origins is that patients with CAA/CAS have purely conductive hearing

Department of Otolaryngology-Head and Neck Surgery, University of Virginia School of Medicine, University of Virginia Department of Otolaryngology, Box 800713, Charlottesville, VA, USA
* Corresponding author.
E-mail address: bwk2n@uvahealth.org

Otolaryngol Clin N Am 56 (2023) 933–948
https://doi.org/10.1016/j.otc.2023.06.007
0030-6665/23/© 2023 Elsevier Inc. All rights reserved.

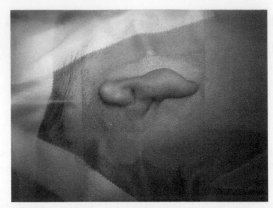

Fig. 1. Classic Grade III microtia with complete atresia of the external auditory canal, right ear.

loss with preserved cochlear function, which informs their prognosis and options for hearing habilitation.

CAA occurs in 1 in 10,000 to 20,000 live births, is 3 times more likely unilateral than bilateral, occurs more often in males, and affects the right ear more often than the left.[1–7] *Aural atresia* refers not only to the failure of the ear canal to develop, but also to some malformation or underdevelopment of the middle ear space and ossicles. Rarely, CAA can be seen in patients with a normal pinna (generally associated with mutations in chromosome 18q[8]), but in general, a more severe external deformity implies a more severe middle ear abnormality.[9]

Hearing habilitation in patients with CAA/CAS can take many forms, both surgical and non-surgical, with and without the use of technology. Although techniques of canalplasty, meatoplasty, tympanoplasty, and ossiculoplasty have improved considerably over the years, surgical correction of CAA remains one of the more challenging operations performed by otologists. This article reviews the evaluation, management, and options for hearing habilitation in patients with congenital anomalies of the ear canal – CAA, CAS, and Type I branchial cleft anomalies.

EMBRYOLOGY/ANATOMY

Understanding the normal embryologic development of the external ear and ear canal are critical for the provider treating congenital anomalies of the outer and middle ear.

The auricle develops from small mounds of epithelium, the hillocks of His, formed from the first and second branchial arches on the side of the embryo. The auricle is developed by the 3rd month of gestation and aberrations within the first 6 weeks of gestation result in microtia. Preauricular pits or sinuses form superior to the tragus and are caused by incomplete fusion of the epithelium of the hillocks resulting in trapped epithelium and an inclusion cyst.

The external auditory canal is derived from the ectoderm of the first branchial cleft. During the second month of gestation, epithelium from this cleft migrates medially as a solid core of tissue which will eventually canalize to form the EAC. The EAC is fully canalized by the 7th month of gestation. Proper formation of the EAC separates the temporomandibular joint (TMJ) anteriorly from the mastoid posteriorly. Further development of the mastoid in normal embryogenesis orients the middle ear and facial nerve in the expected locations. Therefore, in CAA, the TMJ is relatively posterior to its normal location, and the distance between the TMJ and the mastoid tip is decreased.[10]

Commonly, the extent of auricular malformation correlates with the extent of the middle ear malformation, such that milder forms of microtia indicate more developed middle ear structures.[9]

Type I branchial cleft cysts arise from a redundancy, or duplication, of the ectodermal migration of the first branchial arch. Work Type I cysts involve the EAC and are ectodermal only, while Type II cysts involve ectodermal and mesodermal (cartilage) components and often extend to the parotid gland and facial nerve lying inferior to the tragus or in the superior neck.[11]

The first branchial pouch contains endodermal tissue and grows outwardly from the foregut to form the Eustachian tube and middle ear space. The first branchial pouch medially and the first branchial cleft laterally meet at what will become the tympanic membrane, thus explaining the tissue layers of the tympanic membrane with squamous epithelium (ectoderm) laterally and continuous with the EAC, and mucosa (endoderm) lining the medial layer, continuous with the middle ear space. The middle ear ossicles also derive from the first and second branchial arches: the head and neck of the malleus as well as the incus body are formed from Meckel's cartilage, a first branchial arch structure. The long process of the incus and the malleus handle are formed from Reichert's cartilage, a second branchial arch derivative. Reichert's cartilage also forms the stapes suprastructure, while the footplate is derived from both the second arch and the otic placode. Although the malleus head and incus body (first arch) are universally fused and malformed in CAA, the stapes (second arch) are usually normal due to their separate embryonic origins.[4,12] The ossicles are fully formed by the fourth month of gestation. The course of the facial nerve, a second branchial arch derivative, is highly dependent on the development of the surrounding middle ear and mastoid cavities.[13,14] As a result, the facial nerve in CAA courses more anterolaterally from the second genu into the mastoid segment.[13]

TYPE 1 BRANCHIAL CLEFT CYSTS

Branchial cleft anomalies are the most common congenital cervical cystic lesions. Type 1 branchial cleft anomalies are significantly less common than the more common Type 2 branchial cleft anomaly. It is estimated that Type 1 branchial cleft cysts account for less than 10% of all branchial cleft anomalies.[15] When evaluating these lesions, it is important to distinguish between sinus, fistula, and cyst based on their communication (or lack thereof) with surfaces or spaces. Type 1 branchial cleft cysts are classified as either Work type 1 or Work type 2.[11] Work type 1 branchial cleft anomalies may fistulize to the EAC causing repeated episodes of otorrhea/otitis externa, seemingly of unclear etiology. While extremely rare, there are case reports in the literature of coexisting type 1 branchial cleft lesions and microtia, CAA, and congenital cholesteatoma (**Figs. 2** and **3**).[16–18] The anatomy and structural relationships can be quite complex in this region, and a thorough knowledge of the lesion, its extent, and its relationship to surrounding structures including the facial nerve is essential for surgical planning.

Diagnosis/Workup

A full history and physical exam should be obtained with emphasis on the time course and clinical characteristics of the lesion in question. Often, these lesions will fluctuate in size and may intermittently drain or become superinfected, requiring antibiotic therapy. Communication with the EAC may cause otorrhea. In this scenario, the clinician should have a high index of suspicion and look for a fistulous tract along the anterior canal wall; drainage may be expressed into the EAC with pressure over the parotid gland.

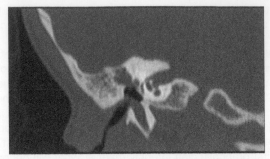

Fig. 2. Coronal CT scan of patient with right congenital aural stenosis and first branchial arch sinus. The sinus tract coursed inferiorly into the upper neck ending in a pit in the neck skin.

If a type 1 branchial cleft anomaly is suspected, imaging is indicated to fully characterize the lesion and its relationship to relevant anatomic structures such as the EAC, parotid gland, and facial nerve (retromandibular vein as the radiographic landmark). While ultrasound may be the first-line imaging modality, it lacks adequate anatomic resolution for this goal. Therefore, computed tomography (CT) is the optimal modality for a more detailed evaluation due to superior spatial resolution and the ability for most children to tolerate the exam (see **Fig. 2**). Magnetic resonance imaging (MRI) has excellent soft tissue resolution; however, most children will have difficulty tolerating the duration of an MRI without sedation. Both CT and MRI have high sensitivity (93% and 89% respectively) in the diagnosis of branchial cleft cysts.[19] Incisional biopsy is not recommended as it will violate tissue planes making complete resection more difficult in the future.

Treatment

As with other branchial cleft anomalies and congenital neck masses, the definitive treatment for type 1 branchial cleft cysts is complete surgical excision (see **Fig. 3**). The extent of the lesion on preoperative imaging will dictate the surgical approach, which will involve the dissection of the preauricular soft tissues. In some cases (eg, Work type II cysts), superficial parotidectomy with facial nerve dissection may be required. Intraoperative facial nerve monitoring is highly recommended. Acutely inflamed or infected lesions should be first treated with broad-spectrum antibiotics to quell the infection before surgical excision.

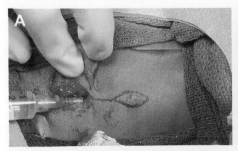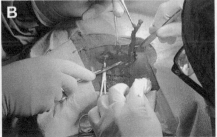

Fig. 3. Intraoperative canalization (A) of the postauricular and neck sinus and subsequent dissection of the fistulous tract (B).

Outcomes

Due to the rarity of first branchial cleft anomalies, there is little data reported in the literature regarding outcomes. A NSQIP analysis established the safety of branchial cleft lesion excision in a large population of children and adults; however, the study did not distinguish between first and second branchial cleft anomalies.[20] Magdy and colleagues reported 18 cases of type 1 branchial cleft cyst excisions, half classified as Work type 1 and half were Work type 2 cysts. 11/18 patients required superficial parotidectomy with facial nerve dissection to ensure complete excision. Two patients had a temporary lower division facial nerve weakness, and all patients recovered to normal facial nerve function within 2 months postoperatively. No data were reported on recurrence rate.[21] Triglia and colleagues reported on 39 patients with first branchial cleft cyst excisions with excellent outcomes and no recurrences reported.[22]

CONGENITAL AURAL ATRESIA
Presentation/Workup

CAA is usually recognized at birth due to its association with microtia (see **Fig. 1**) or due to failure of the newborn hearing screening. Cochlear function in both the atretic and nonatretic ear is most often normal and should be investigated with auditory brainstem response (ABR) testing within the first 3 months of life. ABR testing generally reveals normal bone conduction thresholds with a 50 to 65 dB conductive hearing loss. In the child with unilateral CAA, the normally developed ear usually shows normal hearing, but it is very important to do the ABR test to confirm normal hearing and to reassure parents – normal hearing in one ear is sufficient for normal speech and language development. The clinician must also evaluate the patient for syndromic features: CAA is seen in Goldenhar syndrome/hemifacial microsomia, Treacher Collins syndrome, Crouzon syndrome, Down syndrome (usually EAC stenosis and not complete atresia), and Pierre Robin sequence. Children with such syndromes may also have airway and feeding difficulties which should be recognized and addressed. CT scanning during infancy is not advised.

Treatment Options

Once ABR thresholds have been obtained and hearing status elucidated, parents can be counseled on the options for hearing habilitation, including observation with serial monitoring of the hearing in children with unilateral CAA (testing [ABR or behavioral testing in the booth] every 6 months for the first 2 years of life and then yearly if thresholds remain stable) or bone-conducting hearing devices. A bone conductor on a softband or hardband worn around the head with the processor against the bone of the skull or the processor attached to an adhesive worn behind the ear (AD-HEAR; MED-EL, Innsbruck, Austria) can be offered. Cartilage-conducting hearing devices are being tested in Japan and show some promise.[23] Parents of children with bilateral CAA with normal bone conduction thresholds on ABR are strongly encouraged to place a bone conductor (even bilateral bone conductors[24]) on their child to support normal speech and language development. Ideally, the bone conductor should be fit by an audiologist within the first 3 to 6 months of life.

The benefits of a bone-conducting hearing device in the child with unilateral CAA are less clear. While the bone conductor certainly stimulates central auditory pathways, even without the bone conductor, the child's central auditory pathways are stimulated when the child coos, babbles, speaks, or cries. The child with unilateral CAA is expected to enjoy normal receptive and expressive speech and language development. The more subtle disabilities associated with unilateral hearing loss include difficulty hearing in background noise and poor sound localization. Bone conductors may slightly improve a child's ability to hear in background noise, but they do not aid in sound localization despite relatively high patient satisfaction.[24–26] The decision to place a bone conductor on a child with unilateral conductive hearing loss secondary to CAA is the decision of the family in discussion with the audiologist and physician. Children with unilateral CAA do not show the same disabilities – grade retention, behavioral problems – that children with unilateral sensorineural hearing loss do.[27] Therefore, bone conductors in this setting should never be discouraged, but parents should not be castigated for not having their child wear the bone conductor all day. Many children with unilateral CAA do not adopt these devices or even abandon them after early use. Early placement (before the child develops the motor control to remove the bone conductor) does lead to early acceptance, but, despite anecdotal evidence, no long-term study has shown clear benefit to the use of a bone conductor in unilateral CAA.

For children 5 and older, parents can consider the surgically implanted, osseointe-grated bone conducting devices (OIBCDs); OIBCDs are not FDA approved for children under 5. These devices come as a titanium implant drilled into the bone of the skull attached to a percutaneous abutment (BAHA Connect and Ponto, Cochlear Americas; Lone Tree, CO). Alternatively, transcutaneous systems offer a magnetic plate attached to the same titanium implant (BAHA Attract, Cochlear Americas; Lone Tree, CO). Transcutaneous systems in which the transducer attaches directly to the implant in the bone give improved sound conduction and are approved for children over 12 (BAHA Osia, Cochlear Americas; Lone Tree, CO; Bonebridge, MED-EL, Innsbruck, Austria).

The percutaneous systems offer better sound conduction and a more secure (pro-cessor "snaps" on to the abutment) attachment at the expense of inflammatory skin issues in many patients. This inflammation can often be controlled with topical therapy (temovate steroid cream is helpful), but some patients with persistent inflammation elect to transition to the transcutaneous system. The transcutaneous systems obviate the skin issues seen with the percutaneous systems at the expense of slightly less effi-cient sound conduction (slightly worse hearing) as the sound energy must pass across the skin and subcutaneous tissue to the magnet at the implant. The magnet may also be less secure than the percutaneous implant in an active child on the playground. In the child with unrepaired microtia, placing the OIBCD far enough posteriorly to allow the microtia surgeon pristine tissue for the microtia repair is critical.

Other resources short of a bone conducting hearing device can be utilized and should be discussed to aid the child with CAA (unilateral or bilateral) in language devel-opment and in the classroom. Preferential seating in class, speech therapy, Individu-alized Education Plans (IEPs or 504(c) plans), and FM systems can set the child up for success in the classroom. Clinicians should encourage parents to look into these re-sources within the school system.[27]

Parents of children with CAA should be counseled about the long-term options for rehabilitating the atretic ear(s). Options include observation (if unilateral), microtia repair without atresia surgery, microtia repair with the placement of an OIBCD, or microtia repair with atresia surgery. If the parents are interested in CAA repair, high-resolution CT scan, ideally with less than 1 mm slice thickness, is obtained to deter-mine surgical candidacy (**Fig. 4**). As atresia surgery is not recommended until age 5 or 6 at the earliest, there is no need for imaging prior to this age. The timing of CAA repair also depends on the planned technique for microtia repair. Options for microtia repair include a prosthetic ear attached with medical tape or osseointegrated titanium implants (Vistafix; Cochlear Americas, Lone Tree, CO), repair with autologous rib

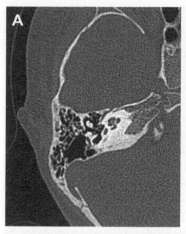
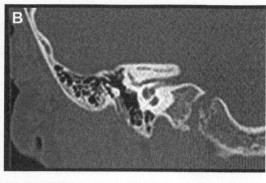

Fig. 4. Axial (A) and coronal (B) CT scan of a good candidate for atresia repair surgery.

cartilage,[28] or implanted porous polyethylene (Medpor; Stryker, Kalamazoo, MI).[29,30] Microtia repair with autologous rib cartilage is performed prior to CAA repair to maximize tissue bed vascular supply for the cartilage graft. The opposite is true with Medpor repair: atresia surgery precedes microtia repair to minimize the risk of an exposed implant.

Classification/Grading Systems

Several classification systems based on high-resolution CT imaging have been proposed, with the intent of predicting the best candidates for surgical repair of CAA. The De la Cruz classification system assesses mastoid pneumatization, inner ear anatomy, and the relationship between the facial nerve and oval window (**Table 1**).[7] The system classifies malformations as either minor or major, with minor malformations treated as surgical candidates and major malformations treated as candidates for bone conducting devices.

The most widely used system is the Jahrsdoerfer grading system which uses a 10-point scale, a point given to each of 8 anatomic structures and two points to the stapes bone; higher scores indicate more normal anatomy, and patients have a greater chance of enjoying normal or near-normal hearing with surgery. Lower scores indicate more severe anomalies and may not be offered surgery (**Tables 2** and **3**).[31,32] Ideal candidates for CAA repair have scores of 8 or greater with 80% to 90% of these

Table 1	
De La Cruz classification of congenital aural atresia	
Minor Malformations	**Major Malformations**
Normal mastoid pneumatization	Poor pneumatization
Normal oval window and stapes footplate	Abnormal or absent oval window and footplate
Good facial nerve and footplate relationship	Abnormal course of the facial nerve
Normal inner ear	Abnormalities of the inner ear

Adapted from De la Cruz A, Linthicum FH, Jr., Luxford WM. Congenital atresia of the external auditory canal. *Laryngoscope.* Apr 1985;95(4):421

Table 2
Jahrsdoerfer grading system for surgery of congenital aural atresia

Parameter	Points
Stapes present	2
Oval window open	1
Middle ear space	1
Facial nerve	1
Malleus/Incus complex	1
Mastoid pneumatization	1
Incus-stapes connection	1
Round window	1
Appearance of external ear	1
Total	10

Adapted from Jahrsdoerfer RA, Yeakley JW, Aguilar EA, Cole RR, Gray LC. Grading system for the selection of patients with congenital aural atresia. *AmJOtol*. Jan 1992;13(1):6.

patients achieving a postoperative speech reception threshold (SRT) of 30 dB HL or below.[32] A score of 7 indicates a fair candidate, while scores of 6 or less are considered poor candidates. Several studies have validated the use of this grading system and have identified finer anatomic details to predict better hearing outcomes, including larger middle ear volume, incudostapedial joint angle less than 120^0, and better preoperative hearing.[32–36]

Operative Technique

A thorough discussion of surgical technique in CAA repair is beyond the scope of this article (for a full step by step approach, see Kesser and Goddard[37]), but a more general review is offered.

The operation essentially consists of 6 steps: approach, drilling the canal, harvesting the skin graft, meatoplasty, placing the eardrum graft, and placing the skin graft. Meticulous technique at each step of the operation is necessary for an optimal outcome. Facial nerve monitoring is a necessity.

With the patient supine and after preparing the surgical site, an incision is made behind the rib graft reconstructed auricle or behind the auricular remnant if the family has chosen Medpor reconstruction (before the Medpor implant is placed). Temporalis fascia is harvested, and mastoid periosteal incisions are made along the linea

Table 3
Interpretation of rating for surgery of congenital aural atresia

Rating	Type of Candidate
10	Excellent
9	Very good
8	Good
7	Fair
6	Marginal
5 or less	Poor

Adapted from Jahrsdoerfer RA, Yeakley JW, Aguilar EA, Cole RR, Gray LC. Grading system for the selection of patients with congenital aural atresia. AmJOtol. Jan 1992;13(1):6.

temporalis and anteriorly, along the glenoid fossa down to the mastoid tip. The peri-osteum is reflected posteriorly, and the periosteum is further elevated to identify the glenoid fossa.

Drilling is performed anterosuperiorly, between the linea temporalis and the glenoid fossa. As the drilling proceeds medially, the tegmen is identified superiorly and fol-lowed medially to open into the epitympanum. The ossicular chain is identified and, using progressively smaller diamond drill burrs, the chain is freed from the surrounding atretic bone. Bony pieces are fractured away from the chain with a dental excavator. Ligamentous attachments are incised to liberate the chain from the inferior aspect of the atretic plate (**Fig. 5**). Special attention is paid while drilling inferiorly as the facial nerve may take an abnormal course through this area. The ossicular chain is exposed circumferentially and is gently palpated to ensure good mobility.

A very thin (0.006 inch thickness) split-thickness skin graft is harvested from the pre-viously prepared upper arm or thigh, measuring roughly 5 cm × 5 cm. The graft is trimmed and the medial edge is notched; 5 "tabs" are thus created on what will become the medial skin graft overlying the neo-tympanic membrane.

Meatoplasty is next performed prior to completing reconstruction. Meatoplasty technique will depend on the microtia repair (for details, see Kesser and Goddard[37]). Assuming good mobility and continuity of the ossicular chain, eardrum reconstruction is then performed with the temporalis fascia graft, which is laid over and "tucked" around the ossicular chain (**Fig. 6**). The skin graft is then brought into the field and delivered into the neo-ear canal. The 5 tabs of the graft are laid sequentially to cover the neo-eardrum. The graft is unfurled to cover all exposed bone of the neo-canal (**Fig. 7**).

Once the graft is appropriately positioned, a silastic disc is placed medially over the fascia and skin graft; ear wicks are trimmed to $^3/_4$ length, placed into the medial canal, and hydrated with antibiotic solution. The lateral skin graft is delivered through the meatus and sutured to the native skin of the concha with rib graft repair, and to the native skin of the postauricular incision in the pre-Medpor repair. More ear wicks are placed to fill the lateral canal. The postauricular incision is closed.

A compressive headwrap is placed and removed on the first postoperative day. The family is instructed on the use of ointment-coated cotton balls in the meatus to maintain a dry canal. The otowicks and silastic disc are removed 7–10 days after surgery. The ear is debrided 6–8 weeks after surgery, and the first audiogram is obtained. Routine maintenance of a well-epithelialized canal will be necessary every 6–12 months.

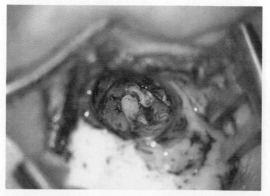

Fig. 5. Drilled right ear canal centered at the malleus-incus complex. Note the fused malleus-incus, incudostapedial joint, and facial nerve.

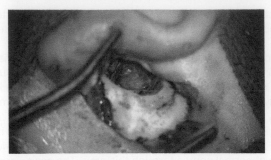

Fig. 6. Temporalis fascia graft in place as neo-tympanic membrane, right ear. Note malleus-incus complex seen through the fascia graft.

Outcomes

Primary goals of atresia surgery are twofold: (1) a clean, dry, skin-lined ear canal, and (2) improvement in air conduction thresholds. Complications of atresia surgery include postoperative stenosis, otorrhea (generally secondary to loss of the skin graft and mucosalization of the medial canal), no improvement in hearing or loss of hearing gains over time, sensorineural hearing loss (rare), and facial nerve injury (very rare[38]).[39] Early studies of hearing outcomes suffered from too short follow-up – only 1 to 3 months after surgery. More recent studies have examined long-term outcomes and show 50% to 75% of patients maintain good hearing (Puretone average [PTA] $\leq$ 30 dB HL) at least 1 year after surgery (**Table 4**). With a mean follow-up of 4.4 years, Imbery and colleagues showed a loss of 8.2 dB over time, with a final gain of 22.2 dB and a final PTA of 37.3 dB HL.[40] As noted above, factors related to improved hearing outcome include middle ear volume,[35] incudostapedial joint angle,[33] preoperative hearing level,[36] and others.[41]

When comparing atresia surgery to OIBCDs, OIBCDs are the clear winner when it comes to ultimate hearing gain, predictability, and final aided PTA.[42–44] However, sound localization,[45] hearing in noise,[46,47] and binaural processing[48,49] may be better with atresia surgery, even if aided with a conventional hearing aid. Percutaneous OIBCDs have issues with skin inflammation/granulation, skin overgrowth, failure of osseointegration, and loosening of the abutment, but do give predictable, reliable sound fidelity to children with conductive hearing loss. Transcutaneous OIBCDs have a less secure attachment to the microphone/processor and less sound fidelity.

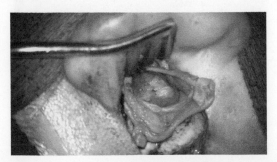

Fig. 7. Split thickness skin graft placed covering the temporalis fascia graft medially and extending up onto the bony canal covering all bony surfaces, right ear.

Table 4
Summary of long-term (>12 mo) hearing outcomes in CAA surgery

Authors	Number of Ears	Follow-up (mos.)	Hearing Outcome
Imbery et al.[40] 2020	138	> 12 (mean 52.8)	22.2 dB gain 64% PTA ≤ 30 dB
Memari et al.[54] 2012	33	12	64% ABG < 30 dB
Moon et al.[55] 2012	68	12	48.7% ABG < 30 dB
El-Hoshy et al.[56] 2008	40	12 24 36	75% PTA 30 dB 65% 65%
Patel and Shelton[57] 2007	52	> 12	61% PTA 30 dB
Digoy and Cueva[58] 2006	16	> 12	75% ABG < 30 dB
Chang et al.[59] 2006	100	12 36	22.03 dB gain 18.1 dB gain

The ultimate decision on hearing habilitation in children with conductive hearing loss secondary to congenital anomalies of the ear canal rests with the family, but the clinician who evaluates and treats children with CAA, unilateral or bilateral, must know all available options–their risks and benefits – including the decision to do nothing. Even if no technological intervention is pursued, the physician must also counsel the family on the options of speech therapy, 504(c) plans, preferential seating in class, FM systems, and good rest.[50]

CONGENITAL AURAL STENOSIS

In the setting of a congenitally narrow (≤3 mm) ear canal, two important issues must be addressed: hearing status and the ear canal's ability to self-clean. Aural stenosis is usually seen with a normally developed auricle, so otomicroscopic examination is not only possible but essential. If the tympanic membrane can be seen, the canal generally will be self-cleaning. Even still, newborn hearing screening (NBHS) should be checked and documented, and if there is any question, further testing should be pursued. Developmental anomalies of the middle ear causing conductive hearing loss can certainly be seen with CAS. Otoacoustic emissions and ABR testing with air and bone conduction thresholds should be performed to document audiometric thresholds. If the child has a conductive hearing loss, consideration should be given to the placement of a bone-conducting hearing device as discussed above (essential if bilateral). Imaging, however, is not necessary in the perinatal period.

A canal in which the eardrum cannot be seen, or a pinpoint canal, is a risk factor for trapped skin and ear canal cholesteatoma. 13% of children with CAA have a stenotic ear canal, and among those with a stenotic ear canal, 19% were found to have an ear canal cholesteatoma.[51] 91% of the ears in patients 12 years and older with EAC stenosis of 2 mm or less harbored cholesteatoma.[52] Both sets of authors argue for the early detection of EAC cholesteatoma in the setting of CAS with high-resolution CT at the age of 4 to 5, a bit earlier than the conventional recommendation of 5 to 6 in the patient with CAA (**Fig. 8**).

Interestingly, surgical outcomes (hearing and creation of a clean, dry, well-epithelialized canal) of patients with CAS tend to be better when compared to patients with CAA probably because of the presence of a naturally skin-lined canal and improved middle ear development and anatomy in the CAS patients despite the cholesteatoma.[53]

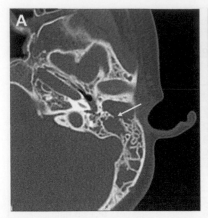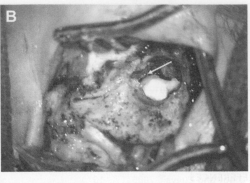

Fig. 8. (*A*) Axial CT scan of left ear canal cholesteatoma that has eroded the posterior canal wall (*arrow*) and has extended into the mastoid cavity. (*B*) Intraoperative picture of same patient. Note erosion of the posterior canal wall (*arrow*) with cholesteatoma extending into drill path to the epitympanum.

SUMMARY

Congenital anomalies of the EAC are rare, and their management requires detailed knowledge of embryology and anatomy as well as nuanced surgical technique. First branchial cleft anomalies and CAA share related embryologic origins. First branchial cleft cysts may be categorized into Work type 1 and Work type 2 and are generally treated with surgical excision. Unilateral CAA is a complex anomaly which may be treated conservatively, with bone conducting devices, or with CAA repair after age 5. Parents and patient should be extensively counseled on the nature of the anomaly and the risks, benefits, and expected outcomes with both surgical and non-surgical interventions. Prior to CAA repair, HRCT should be obtained to verify candidacy using the Jahrsdoerfer grading system. With careful technique, CAA repair can provide patients with long-term hearing improvement. The clinician should have a high index of suspicion for the patient with CAS < 2 mm and pursue HRCT scanning to evaluate for ear canal cholesteatoma.

CLINICS CARE POINTS

- Congenital aural atresia can present as an isolated anomaly, unilateral or bilateral, or in the setting of a craniofacial syndrome; consider possibility of syndromic etiologies of CAA when evaluating the patient with CAA.

- Hearing testing (ABR with air and bone conduction thresholds for both ears) early in the perinatal period is important to document hearing thresholds which inform parent counseling on options for hearing habilitation.

- Consider all options for hearing habilitation:
  ○ Bone conducting technology is a must for children with bilateral CAA to support normal speech and language development
  ○ Bone conducting technology should be considered for children with unilateral CAA; benefits are unclear.
  ○ In select candidates, atresia repair can provide improved hearing with a clean, dry, epithelialized ear canal.

- First branchial cleft cyst or sinus is rare; high index of suspicion is needed to diagnose along with high resolution CT.

- Congenital aural stenosis (CAS) is a rare condition, and hearing testing should be similar to that in children with CAA. Early (age 4–5) CT imaging is recommended in the setting of a canal <2 mm or pinpoint canal to evaluate for trapped skin/ear canal cholesteatoma.

DISCLOSURE

The authors have nothing to disclose.

REFERENCES

1. Gill NW. Congenital atresia of the ear. A review of the surgical findings in 83 cases. J Laryngol Otol 1969;83(6):551–87.
2. Mehra YN, Dubey SP, Mann SB, et al. Correlation between high-resolution computed tomography and surgical findings in congenital aural atresia. Arch Otolaryngol Head Neck Surg 1988;114(2):137–41.
3. Kelemen GM. Aural participation in congenital malformations of the organism. Acta Otolaryngol Suppl 1974;321:1–35.
4. House HP. Management of congenital ear canal atresia. Laryngoscope 1953; 63(10):916–46.
5. Hiraide F, Nomura Y, Nakamura K. Histopathology of atresia auris congenita. J Laryngol Otol 1974;88(12):1249–56.
6. Granstrom G, Tjellstrom A. The bone-anchored hearing aid (BAHA) in children with auricular malformations. Ear Nose Throat J 1997;76(4):238–40.
7. De la Cruz A, Linthicum FH Jr, Luxford WM. Congenital atresia of the external auditory canal. Laryngoscope 1985;95(4):421–7.
8. Cody JD, Sebold C, Heard P, et al. Consequences of chromsome18q deletions. AmJMedGenetCSeminMedGenet 2015;169(3):265.
9. Kountakis SE, Helidonis E, Jahrsdoerfer RA. Microtia grade as an indicator of middle ear development in aural atresia. Arch Otolaryngol Head Neck Surg 1995;121(8):885.
10. Jahrsdoerfer RA, Garcia ET, Yeakley JW, et al. Surface contour three-dimensional imaging in congenital aural atresia. Arch Otolaryngol Head Neck Surg 1993; 119(1):95–9.
11. Work W. Newer concepts of first branchial cleft defects. Laryngoscope 1972;82: 1581–93.
12. Ombredanne M. [Congenital absence of the round window in certain minor aplasias. Further cases]. Ann Otolaryngol Chir Cervicofac 1968;85(5):369–78. Absence congenitale de fenetre ronde dans certaines aplasies mineures. Nouveaux cas.
13. Savic D, Jasovic A, Djeric D. The relations of the mastoid segment of the facial canal to surrounding structures in congenital middle ear malformations. Int J Pediatr Otorhinolaryngol 1989;18(1):13–9.
14. Van de Water TR, Maderson PF, Jaskoll TF. The morphogenesis of the middle and external ear. Birth Defects Orig Artic Ser 1980;16(4):147–80.
15. D'Souza AR, Uppal HS, De R, et al. Updating concepts of first branchial cleft defects: a literature review. Int J Pediatr Otorhinolaryngol 2002;62(2):103–9.
16. Banakis Hartl RM, Said S, Mann SE. Bilateral Ear Canal Cholesteatoma with Underlying Type I First Branchial Cleft Anomalies. Ann Otol Rhinol Laryngol 2019; 128(4):360–4.

17. Jakubikova J, Stanik R, Stanikova A. Malformations of the first branchial cleft: duplication of the external auditory canal. Int J Pediatr Otorhinolaryngol 2005; 69(2):255–61.

18. Yalcin S, Karlidag T, Kaygusuz I, et al. First branchial cleft sinus presenting with cholesteatoma and external auditory canal atresia. Int J Pediatr Otorhinolaryngol 2003;67(7):811–4.

19. Pupic-Bakrac J, Skitarelic N, Novakovic J, et al. Patho-Anatomic Spectrum of Branchial Cleft Anomalies: Proposal of Novel Classification System. J Oral Maxillofac Surg 2022;80(2):341–8.

20. Moroco AE, Saadi RA, Patel VA, et al. Postoperative Outcomes of Branchial Cleft Cyst Excision in Children and Adults: An NSQIP Analysis. Otolaryngol Head Neck Surg 2020;162(6):959–68.

21. Magdy EA, Ashram YA. First branchial cleft anomalies: presentation, variability and safe surgical management. Eur Arch Oto-Rhino-Laryngol 2013;270(6): 1917–25.

22. Triglia JM, Nicollas R, Ducroz V, et al. First branchial cleft anomalies: a study of 39 cases and a review of the literature. Arch Otolaryngol Head Neck Surg 1998; 124(3):291–5.

23. Sakie Akasaka TN, Hosoi Hiroshi, Saito Osamu, et al. Benefits of Cartilage Conduction Hearing Aids for Speech Perception in Unilateral Aural Atresia. Audiol Res 2021;11(2):284–90.

24. Priwin C, Jonsson R, Hultcrantz M, et al. BAHA in children and adolescents with unilateral or bilateral conductive hearing loss: a study of outcome. Int J Pediatr Otorhinolaryngol 2007;71(1):135.

25. Kunst SJ, Leijendeckers JM, Mylanus EA, et al. Bone-anchored hearing aid system application for unilateral congenital conductive hearing impairment: audiometric results. Otol Neurotol 2008;29(1):2.

26. Danhauer JL, Johnson CE, Mixon M. Does the evidence support use of the Baha implant system (Baha) in patients with congenital unilateral aural atresia? J Am Acad Audiol 2010;21(4):274–86.

27. Kesser BW, Krook K, Gray LC. Impact of unilateral conductive hearing loss due to aural atresia on academic performance in children. Laryngoscope. Sep 2013; 123(9):2270.

28. Brent B. Microtia repair with rib cartilage grafts: a review of personal experience with 1000 cases. Clin Plast Surg 2002;29(2):257.

29. Reinisch JF, Lewin S. Ear reconstruction using a porous polyethylene framework and temporoparietal fascia flap. Facial Plast Surg 2009;25(3):181.

30. Romo T 3rd, Presti PM, Yalamanchili HR. Medpor alternative for microtia repair. Facial Plastic Surgery Clinics of North America 2006;14(2):129.

31. Jahrsdoerfer RA, Yeakley JW, Aguilar EA, et al. Grading system for the selection of patients with congenital aural atresia. Am J Otol 1992;13(1):6.

32. Shonka DC Jr, Livingston WJ 3rd, Kesser BW. The Jahrsdoerfer grading scale in surgery to repair congenital aural atresia. Arch Otolaryngol Head Neck Surg 2008;134(8):873.

33. Kim DW, Lee JH, Song JJ, et al. Continuity of the incudostapedial joint: a novel prognostic factor in postoperative hearing outcomes in congenital aural atresia. Acta Otolaryngol 2011;131(7):701.

34. Oliver ER, Lambert PR, Rumboldt Z, et al. Middle ear dimensions in congenital aural atresia and hearing outcomes after atresiaplasty. Otol Neurotol 2010; 31(6):946.

35. Imbery TE, Maldonado M, Mukherjee S, et al. Relationship Between Middle Ear Volume and Long-term Audiological Outcomes in Congenital Aural Atresia Repair. Otol Neurotol 2019;40(6):782–8.

36. Nicholas BD, Krook KA, Gray LC, et al. Does preoperative hearing predict post-operative hearing in patients undergoing primary aural atresia repair? Otol Neurotol 2012;33(6):1002.

37. Kesser B, Goddard J. Congenital Malformation of the External Auditory Canal and Middle Ear. In: Brackman D, Shelton C, Arriaga M, editors. Otologic surgery. 5th edition. Philadelphia, PA: Elsevier; 2023. p. 43–61, chap 4.

38. Jahrsdoerfer RA, Lambert PR. Facial nerve injury in congenital aural atresia surgery. Am J Otol 1998;19(3):283.

39. Oliver ER, Hughley BB, Shonka DC, et al. Revision aural atresia surgery: indications and outcomes. Otol Neurotol 2011;32(2):252.

40. Imbery TE, Gray L, Champaloux E, et al. Long-term Audiometric Outcomes After Atresiaplasty for Congenital Aural Atresia. Otol Neurotol 2020;41(3):371–8.

41. Ahn J, Baek SY, Kim K, et al. Predictive Factors for Hearing Outcomes After Canaloplasty in Patients With Congenital Aural Atresia. Otol Neurotol 2017;38(8):1140.

42. Bouhabel S, Arcand P, Saliba I. Congenital aural atresia: bone-anchored hearing aid vs. external auditory canal reconstruction. Int J Pediatr Otorhinolaryngol 2012;76(2):272.

43. Yellon RF. Atresiaplasty versus BAHA for congenital aural atresia. Laryngoscope 2011;121(1):2.

44. Nadaraja GS, Gurgel RK, Kim J, et al. Hearing outcomes of atresia surgery versus osseointegrated bone conduction device in patients with congenital aural atresia: a systematic review. Otol Neurotol 2013;34(8):1394.

45. Moon IJ, Byun H, Jin SH, et al. Sound localization performance improves after canaloplasty in unilateral congenital aural atresia patients. Otol Neurotol 2014;35(4):639.

46. Byun H, Moon IJ, Woo S-Y, et al. Objective and Subjective Improvement of Hearing in Noise After Surgical Correction of Unilateral Congenital Aural Atresia in Pediatric Patients: A Prospective Study Using the Hearing in Noise Test, the Sound-Spatial-Quality Questionnaire, and the Glasgow Benefit Inventory. Ear Hear 2015;36(4):e183.

47. Gray L, Kesser B, Cole E. Understanding speech in noise after correction of congenital unilateral aural atresia: Effects of age in the emergence of binaural squelch but not in use of head-shadow. Int J Pediatr Otorhinolaryngol 2009;73(9):1281.

48. Kesser BW, Cole ED, Gray LC. Emergence of Binaural Summation After Surgical Correction of Unilateral Congenital Aural Atresia. Otol Neurotol 2016;37(5):499.

49. Wilmington D, Gray L, Jahrsdoerfer R. Binaural processing after corrected congenital unilateral conductive hearing loss. Hear Res 1994;74(1–2):99.

50. Carpenter D, Dougherty W, Sindhar S, et al. Are children with unilateral hearing loss more tired? Int J Pediatr Otorhinolaryngol 2022;155:111075.

51. Casale G, Nicholas BD, Kesser BW. Acquired ear canal cholesteatoma in congenital aural atresia/stenosis. Otol Neurotol 2014;35(8):1474.

52. Cole RR, Jahrsdoerfer RA. The risk of cholesteatoma in congenital aural stenosis. Laryngoscope 1990;100(6):576.

53. Casazza GC, Jonas RH, Kesser BW. Congenital Aural Stenosis With Cholesteatoma. Otol Neurotol 2022;43(3):320–7.

54. Memari F, Mirsalehi M, Jalali A. Congenital aural atresia surgery: transmastoid approach, complications and outcomes. Eur Arch Oto-Rhino-Laryngol 2012; 269(5):1437.
55. Moon IJ, Cho YS, Park J, et al. Long-term stent use can prevent postoperative canal stenosis in patients with congenital aural atresia. Otolaryngol Head Neck Surg 2012;146(4):614.
56. El-Hoshy Z, Abdel-Aziz M, Shabana M. Congenital aural atresia: transmastoid approach; an old technique with good results. Int J Pediatr Otorhinolaryngol 2008;72(7):1047.
57. Patel N, Shelton C. The surgical learning curve in aural atresia surgery. Laryngoscope 2007;117(1):67.
58. Digoy GP, Cueva RA. Congenital aural atresia: review of short- and long-term surgical results. Otol Neurotol 2007;28(1):54.
59. Chang SO, Choi BY, Hur DG. Analysis of the long-term hearing results after the surgical repair of aural atresia. Laryngoscope 2006;116(10):1835.

Dermatologic Conditions of the External Ear
Basics, Updates, and Pearls

Rebecca Leibowitz, BS[a], Jenna E. Koblinski, MD[b],
Latrice M. Hogue, MD[b], Justin T. Cheeley, MD[b],
Travis W. Blalock, MD[b],*

KEYWORDS

- External ear dermatoses • Ear dermatoses • External ear dermatitis • Ear dermatitis

KEY POINTS

- Common dermatoses of the ear including eczema, psoriasis, and vitiligo can be effectively treated with topical steroids and newer non-steroidal medications.
- Genetic evaluation and immunotherapies are becoming more commonly deployed for the assessment and treatment of skin cancers.
- Accurate diagnoses of skin lesions or eruptions may require pathologic evaluation to direct intervention.

INTRODUCTION

Cutaneous disease of the ear comprises a diverse set of presentations, complaints, and causes of morbidity for patients. These findings are common for otolaryngologists and other physicians who interact with patients who have ear complaints. Herein, we seek to provide some timely diagnostic, prognostic, and treatment updates for common auricular diseases.

RASHES
Allergic Contact Dermatitis

Allergic contact dermatitis (ACD) is a type IV delayed hypersensitivity reaction to an allergen that has been in contact with the skin. Some common allergens that may cause ACD in the ear specifically include nickel and other metals found in earrings, hair dyes, ear drops, and certain fragrances found in soaps, shampoos, and lotions.[1,2] The clinical presentation of ACD when it affects the ear includes scaly patches or

[a] Emory University School of Medicine; [b] Department of Dermatology, Emory University School of Medicine, 1525 Clifton Road, Atlanta, GA 30322, USA
* Corresponding author.
E-mail address: travis.w.blalock@emory.edu

Otolaryngol Clin N Am 56 (2023) 949–963
https://doi.org/10.1016/j.otc.2023.05.014
oto.theclinics.com

plaques, erythema, pruritus, and sometimes blistering or crusting of the ear canal, the outer ear, or postauricular sulcus (**Fig. 1**). If chronic, the lesions can become hyperpigmented and lichenified. Treatment typically involves identifying and avoiding the offending allergen. Potential allergens can be identified by taking a thorough history and patch testing, which is an objective measurement of sensitization to allergens.[2] Mild cases can be managed with topical corticosteroids or steroid-sparing agents to reduce inflammation and itching (**Tables 1** and **2**), and oral antihistamines can also be used for itching.[3] In severe cases, oral corticosteroids may be necessary.[2]

Atopic Dermatitis

Atopic dermatitis (AD) is the prototypical eczematous rash in dermatology. It is a common and chronic problem caused by disruptions in the skin's barrier. It is a part of the "atopic triad" and why patients commonly endorse a history or symptoms of seasonal allergies or asthma. AD presents as pruritic ill-defined scaly, erythematous plaques (**Fig. 2**). The more acute form of AD may present with edema and weeping, and the chronic form may evolve into lichen simplex chronicus (thickening of epidermis with accentuation of skin lines). AD may lead to fissures in the skin, which are at-risk for secondary infection (impetigo). Impetigo is classically described as presenting with "honey-colored crust" atop an erythematous, eczematous base (**Fig. 3**). It is important to recognize and treat AD to decrease the risk of infection as well as to provide symptomatic relief for patients.[3]

There are multiple, FDA-approved topical therapies for AD (see **Tables 1** and **2**).[3–5] Topical corticosteroids are the preferred initial treatment of active flares; however, for patients who require long-term management, it may be prudent to initiate a steroid-sparing agent to mitigate long-term effects of topical corticosteroids (see **Table 2**).[3–5] In addition to prescription treatments for AD, liberal moisturization is beneficial to restore the skin's barrier. Patients can be counseled to use a gentle moisturizer at least twice daily. Note that, like topical steroids, moisturizers that are creams or ointments tend to be more efficacious. Applying moisturizers or topical treatment to damp skin after bathing also augments cutaneous water retention. If the patient's AD involves anatomy beyond the ears or becomes extensive, then we would recommend further work-up and treatment, including possible initiation of systemic medications.[3]

For secondary impetiginization of eczematous lesions on the ears, topical mupirocin ointment can be used as can systemic antibiotics based on physician judgment. We

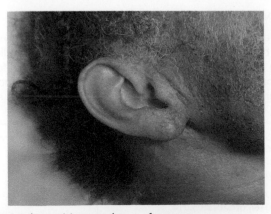

Fig. 1. Allergic contact dermatitis secondary to fragrance.

Table 1
Topical corticosteroids

Name/Strength/Formulation	Steroid Class	Dosing	Adverse Events	Indications
Clobetasol propionate 0.05% cream, ointment, or solution	1 (Ultra high potency)	Twice daily for up to two weeks to thick plaques, then as needed for maintenance. Avoid face, groin, skin folds, normal skin.	Long-term use associated with atrophy, striae, and dyspigmentation.	Allergic/irritant contact dermatitis, atopic dermatitis, discoid lupus erythematosus, psoriasis[a], sarcoidosis, vitiligo
Triamcinolone acetonide 0.1% cream or ointment	3 (High)	Twice daily for up to two weeks, then as needed for maintenance. Avoid face, groin, skin folds, normal skin.	Long-term use associated with atrophy, striae, and dyspigmentation.	Allergic/irritant contact dermatitis[a], atopic dermatitis[a], discoid lupus erythematosus, psoriasis[a], sarcoidosis, seborrheic dermatitis[a], vitiligo
Fluocinolone acetonide 0.01% oil[b]	5 (Medium)	Twice daily for up to two weeks, then as needed for maintenance.	Long-term use associated with atrophy, striae, and dyspigmentation.	Allergic/irritant contact dermatitis, atopic dermatitis[a], discoid lupus erythematosus, psoriasis[a], sarcoidosis, seborrheic dermatitis[a]

[a] Food and Drug Administration-approved indication.
[b] Comes in an ear drop formulation.

Table 2
Steroid-sparing agents

Name/Strength/Formulation	Mechanism of Action	Dosing	Indications
Calcipotriene 0.005% ointment	Vitamin D3 analogue	Twice daily as needed	Psoriasis[a]
Crisaborale 2% ointment	Phosphodiesterase-4 inhibitor	Twice daily as needed	Atopic dermatitis[a], vitiligo[a]
Ketoconazole 2% cream or shampoo (as a wash)	Anti-fungal	Twice daily for 4 weeks or until clinical response noted	Seborrheic dermatitis[a]
Ketoconazole 2% shampoo (as a wash)	Anti-fungal	Two to three times weekly	Seborrheic dermatitis[a]
Pimecrolimus 1% ointment	Calcineurin inhibitor	Twice daily as needed	Allergic/irritant contact dermatitis, atopic dermatitis[a], discoid lupus erythematosus, psoriasis, sarcoidosis, seborrheic dermatitis, vitiligo
Ruxolitinib phosphate 1.5% cream	Janus kinase (JAK) inhibitor	Twice daily as needed. Maximum dose: 60 g per week or 100 g per two weeks.	Atopic dermatitis[a], seborrheic dermatitis, vitiligo[a]
Tacrolimus 0.1% ointment	Calcineurin inhibitor	Twice daily as needed	Allergic/irritant contact dermatitis, atopic dermatitis[a], discoid lupus erythematosus, psoriasis, sarcoidosis, seborrheic dermatitis, vitiligo
Tazorotene 0.05% cream or gel	Acetylene retinoid	Apply once daily in evening as needed	Second-line treatment of psoriasis[a]

[a] FDA-approved indication.

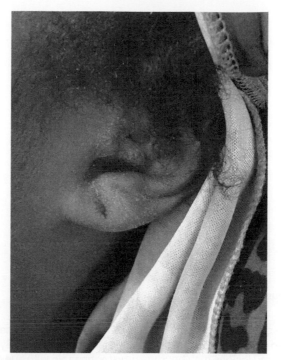

Fig. 2. Atopic dermatitis.

would caution against patients using over-the-counter antibiotic creams or ointments as those often contain common allergens that can then cause secondary ACD and worsening rash.[3] As discussed below with otitis externa, dilute acetic acid has been shown to help treat/prevent progression into otitis externa.[6]

Discoid Lupus Erythematosus

Discoid lupus erythematosus (DLE) is a chronic autoimmune disorder that affects the skin, causing scarring and pigment changes. DLE is a subtype of cutaneous lupus erythematosus characterized by round or oval-shaped patches of scaly, red or pink indurated plaques (**Fig. 4**).[7] These plaques may slowly expand with active inflammation on

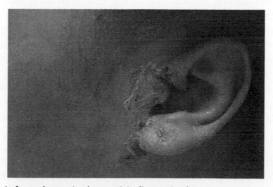

Fig. 3. Secondarily infected atopic dermatitis (impetigo).

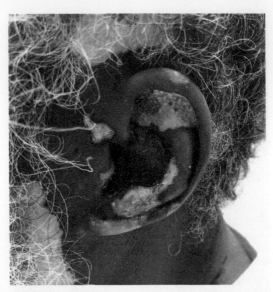

Fig. 4. Discoid lupus erythematosus.

the periphery and scarring or atrophy centrally. DLE can occur on the face, neck, and scalp but may also occur on the ears, especially the conchal bowls. Symptoms include pruritus and pain, and lesions may become more noticeable with sun exposure. Treatment options for DLE aim to reduce inflammation and prevent scarring. Mild cases may be managed with topical corticosteroids or calcineurin inhibitors (see **Tables 1** and **2**), while more severe cases may require systemic medications such as hydroxychloroquine, methotrexate, or mycophenolate mofetil.[3,8] Sun protective measures such as wearing protective clothing and using sunscreen are also important to prevent worsening of the condition. In cases where scarring is severe, cosmetic procedures such as laser therapy or dermabrasion may be considered.[9]

Otitis externa

Otitis externa is an inflammatory infection of the external ear canal that is most commonly caused by bacteria.[10] Clinical presentation of otitis externa includes pain, itching, redness, and swelling in the ear canal, as well as discharge and hearing loss (**Fig. 5**). In severe cases, there may be fever and lymph node swelling in the neck. Risk factors for otitis externa include swimming, use of hearing aids or earplugs, and trauma to the ear canal. People with skin conditions such as eczema, psoriasis, or seborrheic dermatitis may also be at higher risk for otitis externa. Treatment options for otitis externa depend on the severity of the infection. Mild cases can often be treated with topical medications such as acetic acid 2%, aminoglycosides, polymyxin B, and quinolones with and without corticosteroids.[6] More severe infections, including cases involving cellulitis, may require oral antibiotics. In addition, measures like avoiding water exposure and keeping the ear canal dry may help prevent recurrent infections. Furthermore, dilute acetic acid has been shown to help treat/prevent otitis externa.[6]

Psoriasis

Psoriasis is a chronic, commonly pruritic rash that classically presents with well-demarcated, erythematous plaques with thick silvery scale that has a predilection for the scalp, extensor surfaces, and the buttocks. Ear psoriasis may present

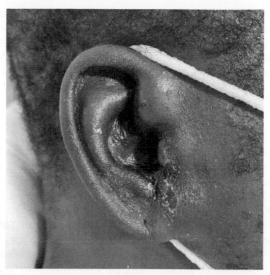

Fig. 5. Otitis externa.

diversely, from post-auricular to conchal bowl to even extension into the external auditory canal (**Fig. 6**). Scalp and ear psoriasis can also be seen as a spectrum with seborrheic dermatitis ("sebopsoriasis") and this may appear as more loose scale without the discrete plaques. Topical treatment of psoriasis is similar to treatment of AD with a short-term focus on topical corticosteroids followed by transitioning to a long-term steroid sparing agent as appropriate (see **Tables 1** and **2**). If the patient's psoriasis involves other areas of the body beyond the ears or the patient endorses arthritic symptoms, then we would recommend assessment to determine whether initiation of systemic medications would be appropriate.[3]

Sarcoidosis

Cutaneous sarcoidosis is present in up to one-third of patients with sarcoidosis and appears most often on the face but may also present on the ear.[3] This granulomatous

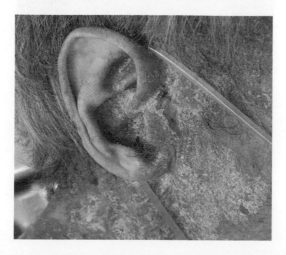

Fig. 6. Psoriasis.

disease classically presents as red-brown to violaceous papules and plaques (**Fig. 7**), but can vary broadly including presenting as a rash. If cutaneous sarcoidosis is suspected, a biopsy should be performed and if the diagnosis is confirmed, then the patient should be referred to pulmonology and rheumatology specialists as well as cardiology and dermatology (as appropriate) for evaluation of systemic disease and further treatment. For localized treatment of sarcoidosis on the ear, either topical or intralesional steroids may be initiated (see **Table 1**).[3]

Seborrheic Dermatitis

Seborrheic dermatitis is a common, chronic dermatitis. It occurs predominantly in areas with active sebaceous glands (such as the scalp, face, ears, and pre-sternal area), which encourages growth of normal skin yeast. The clinical presentation can vary from classic dandruff to thin, pink-yellow patches with "greasy" appearing scale (**Fig. 8**). It can be pruritic.[3] Treatment of seborrheic dermatitis of the ears includes topical corticosteroids and topical anti-fungal medications (see **Tables 1** and **2**).[3,11] There is also some evidence for using topical calcineurin inhibitors as well as topical JAK inhibitors.[4,11,12] In addition to prescription topicals, over-the-counter dandruff shampoos containing selenium sulfide or zinc pyrithione can also be useful and affordable adjuncts. Most commonly, we recommend allowing these shampoos to remain on the scalp for several minutes before washing them off in order to to optimize efficacy.[3]

Vitiligo

Vitiligo is an autoimmune disorder that leads to depigmented macules and patches of skin. It may occur anywhere on the skin, including the ears. In patients with lighter skin tones, it may be difficult to appreciate depigmented lesions, and thus a Wood's lamp can be a useful tool; this will accentuate the depigmented nature of involved skin compared with the patient's normal tone.[3] Localized treatment includes medium- to

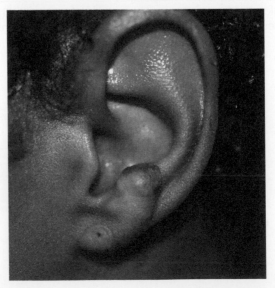

Fig. 7. Sarcoidosis.

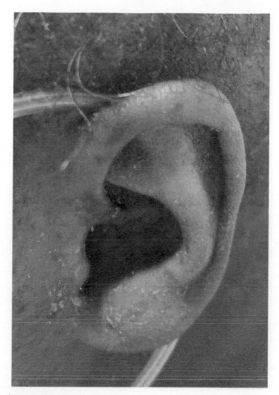

Fig. 8. Seborrheic dermatitis.

high-strength topical corticosteroids (see **Table 1**) as well as a select number of topical steroid-sparing agents (see **Table 2**).[4,13]

BENIGN LESIONS
Keloids

Keloids are benign growths of dense fibroproliferative tissue that can form in areas of previously traumatized skin, such as a cut, burn, or surgical incisions. Keloids are clinically characterized by raised, thickened papules and nodules that extend beyond the boundaries of the original injury site as opposed to hypertrophic scars (**Fig. 9**).[14] They are often associated with itchiness, tenderness, or pain and can cause cosmetic concerns, particularly if they are located on visible areas such as the face, neck, or ears.[15] Keloids are more common in individuals with darker skin types and tend to occur more frequently in certain areas, such as the chest, shoulders, and earlobes. Treatment options for keloids include intralesional injections, surgical excision, cryotherapy, laser therapy, and pressure therapy. Intralesional corticosteroid injections, usually with triamcinolone acetonide, is often used as monotherapy for small keloids. Efficacy can be increased when used in combination with other therapies such as steroid tapes/plasters or intralesional chemotherapeutic agents, such as bleomycin or fluorouracil. Surgical excision of keloids can be performed alone or can be used with adjuvant therapies such as intralesional injections or radiation therapy to minimize recurrence. Cryotherapy and laser therapy can be effective as either monotherapy or in combination with other modalities; however, caution should be taken for concern

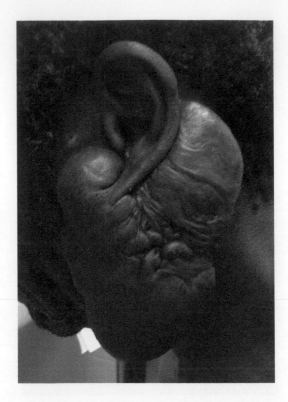

Fig. 9. Keloid.

for dyspigmentation in darker skin types. Keloids are difficult to treat and recurrence rates are high. Management may require a combination of different treatments, a step-wise treatment plan, and close follow-up in order to monitor and/or treat clinical recurrence.[3,16]

Melanocytic Nevi of Ear

Melanocytic nevi of the ear are benign proliferations of melanocytes that develop on the skin of the ear.[17] Clinical presentation of melanocytic nevi can vary depending on the type and anatomic location of the nevus. Some melanocytic nevi are small and flat, while others may be elevated with various colors including brown, black, or pink. Some nevi may also exhibit hair growth. Not uncommonly, some melanocytic nevi of the ear may exhibit clinical features (growth, changes in coloration, ulceration, etc.) that mimic melanoma and thus warrant a biopsy to rule out malignancy. Treatment options for melanocytic nevi of the ear vary based on the size and appearance of the lesion. Small, flat nevi that are not changing and are asymptomatic may not require treatment and simply require serial monitoring, with our without dermoscopy. Treatment options for clinically concerning or symptomtic melanocytic nevi of the ear include surgical excision. Of note treatment of melanocytic nevi is different than treatment of other types of nevi, like epidermal nevi, which may warrant surgical excision, cryotherapy, or even ablative laser therapy.[18]

Verruca Vulgaris

Verrucae vulgaris (warts) are caused by human papillomavirus infection of the epidermis, with the hands, feet, and face as the most common sites of infection.[19]

Although there have been case reports of verrucae occurring in the external auditory canal and on the tympanic membrane, verrucae on the ear are overall relatively rare.[19,20] Gross examination of these lesions reveals clusters of flesh-colored papillomatous nodules with a characteristic cauliflower shape. Although there are many treatments available for verrucae, lesions located in the ear have demonstrated successful responses to liquid nitrogen, surgical excision, intralesional bleomycin, and topical immunomodulatory therapies like imiquimod.[19,20]

PRE-MALIGNANT/MALIGNANT LESIONS
Actinic Keratosis

Actinic keratoses (AKs) are pre-neoplastic lesions formed by the proliferation of dysplastic keratinocytes. They tend to occur in sun exposed areas and have the potential for malignant transformation into non-melanoma skin cancer (NMSC), namely cutaneous squamous cell carcinoma (cSCC).[21] AKs often develop on the ear, with the helical rim as the most common site, and present as poorly defined papules or patches with an erythematous base and rough texture and hyperkeratosis.[22] Malignant transformation to cSCC can be eliminated or delayed with surgical and/or topical treatments. Surgical treatments for AKs include cryosurgery and curettage and electrodessication, while topical treatments include 5-fluorouracil (5-FU), imiquimod, and retinoids. AKs treated with field-directed therapies, such as 5-FU and imiquimod, have been shown to have lower recurrence rates than photodynamic therapy.[21] Many

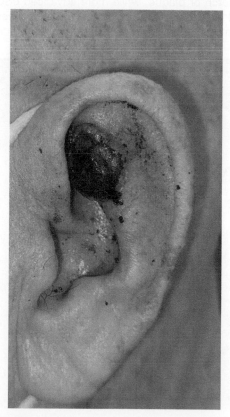

Fig. 10. Basal cell carcinoma.

advocate for lesion-directed therapy for thicker individual hyperkeratotic lesions and a field-therapy approach for less discriminate and multiple thinner hyperkeratotic lesions that commonly populate a larger region.[3,21]

Basal Cell Carcinoma

Basal cell carcinoma (BCC) is the most common malignancy nationwide and accounts for over 90% of skin cancer diagnoses.[23,24] It is also the most common skin cancer of the ear, comprising 20% of ear malignancies overall.[22–24] Moreover, while the majority of ear BCCs arise on helical and periauricular areas, 15% occur in the external auditory canal.[22] Clinically, the lesion is classically described as a flesh-colored papule with a pearly border, surrounding telangiectasias, and central ulceration (**Fig. 10**). Although most BCCs can be adequately treated with standard surgical resection or Mohs micrographic surgery, rare high-risk BCCs may require targeted chemotherapy or immunotherapy, such as smoothened inhibitors (ie, vismodegib) or checkpoint inhibitors.[25,26] Cemiplimab, a PD-1 antibody, was shown to have potent antitumor activity against BCCs, with 31% of patients demonstrating an objective response to therapy in a recent phase II trial.[26]

Cutaneous Squamous Cell Carcinoma

cSCC accounts for up to 20% of NMSC and is responsible for the majority of NMSC-related metastasis and death.[27,28] Its clinical presentation most commonly involves an erythematous scaly patch or plaque, while more advanced cSCC can also present with ulceration (**Fig. 11**). Almost one-quarter of cSCC of the head and neck involve the ear, with most tumors originating on the helix and antihelical margin.[22] Surgical

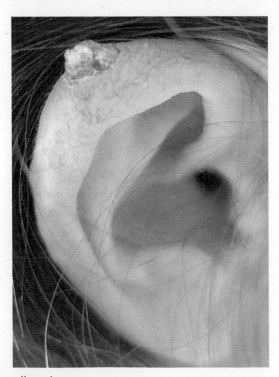

Fig. 11. Squamous cell carcinoma.

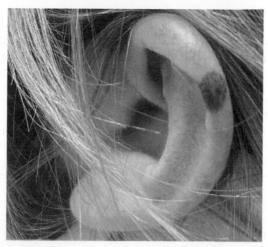

Fig. 12. Melanoma.

resection by standard excision or Mohs surgery currently serves as the gold standard, with Mohs surgery providing higher cure rates and potential for tissue conservation. In more advanced or metastatic disease, tumor-specific gene expression profiles are becoming more commonly used to help manage patient care including when to radiate and how to monitor for recurrence.[29] Additionally, immunotherapy, like the PD-1 inhibitor cemiplimab, is becoming a mainstay in treatment of metastatic disease.[30] How gene expression profiling and immunotherapy will fit within the larger treatment and management landscape in the coming years is quickly evolving.

Melanoma

Melanoma represents the malignant transformation of melanocytes. Although melanoma only accounts for less than 2% of cancer diagnoses, it is responsible for a disproportionately larger percentage of skin cancer mortality.[31] Approximately one-fifth of primary melanomas occur on the head and the neck, with 7–14% located on the peripheral parts of the ear.[8] The clinical presentation of melanoma varies widely; patients often report a hyperpigmented macule, patch, or nodule with asymmetric borders and a history of a change in size or color (**Fig. 12**). Over the last forty years, the incidence of melanoma has continued to increase; however, mortality rates have declined due to the advent of novel systemic therapies, most notably immune checkpoint inhibitors in the recent past.[32] In situ or stage I melanoma is commonly treated with excision alone, while more advanced stages may require adjuvant therapies, such as BRAF, MEK, and c-KIT inhibitors.[33–35]

SUMMARY

Numerous dermatologic conditions can present on the ear and can be challenging to diagnose and manage due to the localized anatomy and varied etiologies. It is essential to obtain a thorough patient history, perform a comprehensive physical examination, and consider biopsy or other diagnostic studies when necessary to establish an accurate diagnosis. Treatment options depend on the specific condition and may include topical and systemic medications, lifestyle modifications, and surgical interventions. Prompt and appropriate management can improve patient outcomes and prevent complications.

CLINICS CARE POINTS

- Secondary impetiginization may occur in association with numerous types of dermatitis, thus warranting consideration of a culture to guide treatment.

- Genetic testing of melanoma as well as non-melanoma skin cancer is becoming more commonplace, though the deployment of such tests will likely require further studies to clarify which situations require them.

- Mohs micrographic surgery remains the current gold standard surgical treatment of cutaneous squamous cell and basal cell carcinoma of the ear due to tissue conservation and superior cure rates.

REFERENCES

1. Garner LA. Contact dermatitis to metals. Dermatol Ther 2004;17(4):321–7.
2. Nassau S, Fonacier L. Allergic contact dermatitis. Med Clin 2020;104(1):61–76.
3. Bolognia J, Schaffer JV, Cerroni L. Dermatology. Fourth ed. Philadelphia, PA: Elsevier; 2018.
4. Shalabi MMK, Garcia B, Coleman K, et al. Janus kinase and tyrosine kinase inhibitors in dermatology: a review of their utilization, safety profile and future applications. Skin therapy letter 2022;27(1):4.
5. Mancuso-Stewart E, Rodger J, Zirwas M. Overview of safety, efficacy, and patient counseling for ruxolitinib in treating atopic dermatitis. Skinmed 2023; 21(1):40–3.
6. Rosenfeld RM, Schwartz SR, Cannon CR, et al. Clinical practice guideline: acute otitis externa. Otolaryngology-head and neck surgery 2014;150(1_suppl): S1–24.
7. Joseph AK, Windsor B, Hynan LS, et al. Discoid lupus erythematosus skin lesion distribution and characteristics in Black patients: a retrospective cohort study. Lupus Sci Med 2021;8(1):1–5.
8. Foulke G, Helm LA, Clebak KT, et al. Autoimmune skin conditions: cutaneous lupus erythematosus. FP essentials (Online) 2023;526:25.
9. Joseph AK, Abbas LF, Chong BF. Treatments for disease damage in cutaneous lupus erythematosus: a narrative review. Dermatol Ther 2021;34(5):e15034, n/a.
10. Jackson EA, Geer K. Acute otitis externa: rapid evidence review. Am Fam Physician 2023;107(2):145–51.
11. Kastarinen H, Oksanen T, Okokon EO, et al. Topical anti-inflammatory agents for seborrhoeic dermatitis of the face or scalp. Cochrane Database Syst Rev 2014; 5(8):CD009446.
12. Pope E, Kowalski E, Tausk F. Topical ruxolitinib in the treatment of refractory facial seborrheic dermatitis. JAAD Case Reports 2022;24:59–60.
13. Sheikh A, Rafique W, Owais R, et al. FDA approves ruxolitinib (opzelura) for vitiligo therapy: a breakthrough in the field of dermatology. Annals of medicine and surgery 2022;81:104499.
14. Berman B, Maderal A, Raphael B. Keloids and hypertrophic scars: pathophysiology, classification, and treatment. Dermatol Surg 2017;43(Suppl 1):S3–18.
15. Walsh LA, Wu E, Pontes D, et al. Keloid treatments: an evidence-based systematic review of recent advances. Syst Rev 2023;12(1):42.
16. Betarbet U, Blalock TW. Keloids: a review of etiology, prevention, and treatment. J Clin Aesthet Dermatol 2020;13(2):33–43.

17. Lim HJ, Kim YT, Choo O-S, et al. Clinical and histological characteristics of melanocytic nevus in external auditory canals and auricles. Eur Arch Oto-Rhino-Laryngol 2013;270(12):3035–42.
18. Rajpal N, Dilorenzo A, Parsa K, et al. Bilateral epidermal nevi in the external auditory canals treated with CO2 laser. Pediatr Dermatol 2020;37(2):388–9.
19. Lee JH, Burm JS, Yang WY, et al. Treatment of verruca vulgaris in both external auditory canals using bleomycin injections. Clinical and experimental otorhinolaryngology 2015;8(3):295–7.
20. Shangkuan W-CMD, Lin M-YMD. Verruca vulgaris of tympanic membrane treated with topical immunotherapy. Am J Otolaryngol 2014;35(2):242–5.
21. Reinehr CPH, Bakos RM. Actinic keratoses: review of clinical, dermoscopic, and therapeutic aspects. Anais brasileiros de dermatología 2019;94(6):637–57.
22. Sand M, Sand D, Brors D, et al. Cutaneous lesions of the external ear. Head Face Med 2008;4(1):2.
23. Kim DP, Kus KJB, Ruiz E. Basal Cell Carcinoma Review. Hematol Oncol Clin North Am 2019;33(1):13–24.
24. Basal Cell and Squamous Cell Carcinoma. Available at: https://www.ucsfhealth.org/conditions/basal-cell-and-squamous-cell-carcinoma. Published 2022. Accessed April 7, 2023.
25. Sekulic A, Migden MR, Oro AE, et al. Efficacy and safety of vismodegib in advanced basal-cell carcinoma. N Engl J Med 2012;366(23):2171–9.
26. Stratigos AJ, Sekulic A, Peris K, et al. Cemiplimab in locally advanced basal cell carcinoma after hedgehog inhibitor therapy: an open-label, multi-centre, single-arm, phase 2 trial. Lancet Oncol 2021;22(6):848–57.
27. Burton KA, Ashack KA, Khachemoune A. Cutaneous squamous cell carcinoma: a review of high-risk and metastatic disease. Am J Clin Dermatol 2016;17(5):491–508.
28. Yanofsky VR, Mercer SE, Phelps RG. Histopathological variants of cutaneous squamous cell carcinoma: a review. Journal of skin cancer 2011;2011:210813.
29. Arron ST, Blalock TW, Guenther JM, et al. Clinical considerations for integrating gene expression profiling into cutaneous squamous cell carcinoma management. J Drugs Dermatol 2021;20(6):5s–s11.
30. Shalhout SZ, Emerick KS, Kaufman HL, et al. Immunotherapy for non-melanoma skin cancer. Curr Oncol Rep 2021;23(11):125.
31. Cancer Facts & Figures 2017. American Cancer Society. Available at: https://www.cancer.org/research/cancer-facts-statistics/all-cancer-facts-figures/cancer-facts-figures-2017.html. Published 2017. Accessed April 7, 2023.
32. Siegel RL, Miller KD, Jemal A. Cancer statistics, 2020. CA: a cancer journal for clinicians 2020;70(1):7–30.
33. Rizos H, Menzies AM, Howie J, et al. BRAF inhibitor resistance mechanisms in metastatic melanoma: spectrum and clinical impact. Clin Cancer Res 2014;20(7):1965–77.
34. Domingues B, Lopes JM, Soares P, et al. Melanoma treatment in review. ImmunoTargets Ther 2018;7:35–49.
35. Treatment of melanoma skin cancer by stage. American Cancer Society. Available at: https://www.cancer.org/cancer/melanoma-skin-cancer/treating/by-stage.html. Published 2022. Accessed April 7, 2023.

Neoplasms of the Ear Canal

Mallory Raymond, MD*

KEYWORDS

- External auditory canal • Neoplasm • Bony • Ceruminous • Cutaneous

KEY POINTS

- Osteoma and exostoses are related in histology, often asymptomatic, diagnosed incidentally and might not require intervention.
- Benign and malignant glandular EAC neoplasms are rare, can present similarly and can share histologic characteristics.
- Squamous cell carcinoma is the most common malignant neoplasm of the EAC and should be considered in patients with unresolving otitis externa or non-healing ulcerative or friable lesions.
- Sleeve resection of the EAC skin has a limited role in the surgical treatment of cutaneous malignancies.

INTRODUCTION

Neoplasms of the EAC can be described by their cell of origin and further divided into lesions arising primarily from within the EAC or involving the EAC secondarily from a separate primary location. Given the histologic components of the EAC, primary neoplasms can be broadly classified into bony, glandular and cutaneous (**Table 1**). Neoplasms that secondarily involve the EAC include metastasis and those arising from within the middle ear, mastoid or jugular foramen. This article will review these classifications, focusing on histopathology, clinical characteristics, prognosis, and management.

Bony

Exostoses are benign generally broad-based rounded bony growths that arise circumferentially as multiple lesions in the medial EAC, often bilateral and symmetric, and consisting of layers of subperiosteal bone containing no bone marrow.[1] Their formation is correlated with cold water exposure and thought to arise due to cold-induced periostitis. Clinical presentation varies with the degree of EAC occlusion and can

Department of Otolaryngology – Head and Neck Surgery, Mayo Clinic Florida, 4500 San Sablo Drive, Jacksonville, FL 32224, USA
* Corresponding.author.
E-mail address: raymond.mallory@mayo.edu

Otolaryngol Clin N Am 56 (2023) 965–976
https://doi.org/10.1016/j.otc.2023.06.003
oto.theclinics.com

Table 1
Neoplasms of the ear canal classified by cell of origin

Bony	
Benign	Osteoma
	Exostoses
Glandular	
Benign	Ceruminous gland adenoma
	Ceruminous pleomorphic adenoma
	Ceruminous syringocystadenoma papilliferum
Malignant	Ceruminous adenoid cystic carcinoma
	Ceruminous adenocarcinoma NOS
	Ceruminous mucoepidermoid carcinoma
Cutaneous	
Benign	Squamous papilloma
	Pilomatrixoma
Malignant	Squamous cell carcinoma
	Basal cell carcinoma
	Melanoma
	Merkel cell carcinoma
Metastatic	Parotid, colorectal, bronchogenic, esophageal adenocarcinomas; small cell, hepatocellular, prostate, renal cell carcinoma
Arising from secondary site	Paraganglioma, sarcoma, schwannoma, hemangioma, Langerhans cell histiocytosis, lymphoma, extramedullary plasmacytoma, leukemia, solitary fibrous tumor

include conductive hearing loss and otitis externa.[2] High resolution computed tomography (CT) of the temporal bone will delineate the depth of bony involvement as well as the presence of any medial cholesteatoma formation. Management includes observation for asymptomatic individuals or exostectomy and canalplasty for symptomatic individuals. A variety of approaches using the drill or osteotome have been described. Advantages of the osteotome include decreased risk of sensorineural hearing loss and postoperative stenosis, while the drill might reduce the risk of tympanic membrane perforation.[2] Preservation of native canal skin is paramount to reducing the risk of stenosis.[3]

Osteomata are benign generally solitary, pedunculated smooth, round lesions arising along the tympanomastoid and tympanosquamous suture line. Histologically they consist of lamellar bone with outer cortical and inner bone marrow spaces, differentiating osteomata from exostoses.[1] Osteomata are often diagnosed incidentally. Most individuals are asymptomatic. For symptomatic individuals, surgical removal can done be via a transcanal or postauricular approach using a drill or osteotome. Preoperative CT imaging can delineate the medial extent of the osteoma and the presence of medial debris (**Fig. 1**). Similar to exostectomy, skin flaps are created with the intention of skin preservation and the bony lesion is drilled to its base. Complete removal of the base is recommended to prevent recurrence.[3]

Glandular

Glandular neoplasms of the EAC are uncommon. Formerly called ceruminomas, they are thought to arise from ceruminous glands, which are concentrated in the lateral membranous portion of the EAC. The World Health Organization (WHO) currently classifies both benign and malignant EAC glandular tumors.[1]

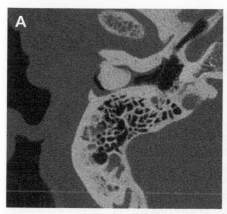
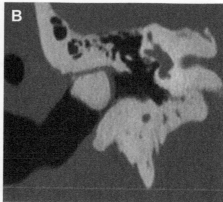

Fig. 1. High resolution CT temporal bone of the right external auditory canal in the axial (*A*) and coronal (*B*) planes demonstrating a large superiorly based osteoma originating from a relatively narrow stalking, causing near complete canal occlusion.

Benign

Benign EAC glandular tumors include ceruminous gland adenoma, ceruminous pleomorphic adenoma and syringocystoma papilliferum. Patients are often asymptomatic but found by otologic exam to have a soft well-circumscribed lesion occupying the membranous EAC, not associated with ulceration or destruction. Rarely are these lesions identified in pediatric patients.[4,5] On imaging, benign lesions will be well-circumscribed with homogeneous enhancement with or without cystic changes and no bony infiltration.[6] Once biopsy confirms the histology, a wide local excision and reconstruction is recommended.

Ceruminous gland adenomas, or more recently termed adenoma not-otherwise-specified (NOS), are the most common benign glandular EAC tumors.[1] They are firm nonencapsulated masses with smooth surfaces and are composed of well-differentiated glandular structures lined by epithelium. The average age of presentation is in the 6th decade.[5,7] There is no sex predilection.

Ceruminous pleomorphic adenoma (CPA) is the second most common EAC benign glandular neoplasm.[7] Tumors are firm, nonencapsulated, and well-circumscribed and are composed of both epithelial and mesenchymal elements, similar to pleomorphic adenomas in the head and neck.[7] Typically, primary neoplasms present as enlarging masses with occlusive and compressive symptoms. There appears to be a slight male predominance, though the average age of presentation is less than that of patients with adenoma NOS.[6]

Ceruminous syringocystadenoma papilliferum (SCAP) is an extremely rare tumor of the EAC with only a few case reports in the literature.[8–12] Tumors can be polypoid, lobulated or ulcerated, containing multiple short, thick papillae.[13] Presenting symptoms are similar to those of other benign EAC neoplasms. Most reported cases were diagnosed in the 7th to 8th decade of life.

Malignant

There is clinical and histologic overlap between benign and malignant EAC glandular tumors, though malignant neoplasms appear to be slightly more common.[13] In descending order of frequency, these include ceruminous adenoid cystic carcinoma, adenocarcinoma NOS, and mucoepidermoid carcinoma.[13] Patients can be asymptomatic or present with canal occlusion, otalgia and facial weakness. Tumors are more likely to ulcerate and exhibit perineural invasion. They can extend through the fissures of Santorini into the parotid gland, into periauricular soft tissue, through the tympanic membrane or into the bony and cartilaginous EAC. Adequate depth of biopsy is needed to distinguish between benign and malignant neoplasms. CT and MRI should be obtained to delineate the extent of invasion.

Ceruminous adenoid cystic carcinoma

The origin cell-type of ceruminous adenoid cystic carcinoma of the EAC is unknown but it shares features with malignant salivary gland tumors. Tumors are unencapsulated, diffusively infiltrative and invasive into deep tissue and perineurium, and made up of monomorphic basaloid cells arranged in tubular, cribriform or solid patterns. The solid pattern carries the worse prognosis.[14,15] Alterations of the MYB transcription factors seen in salivary gland adenoid cystic carcinoma might also occur in ceruminous adenoid cystic carcinoma,[16,17] however tumors that do not stain for MYB might have a worse prognosis.[18]

Ceruminous adenoid cystic carcinoma is approximately twice as common in females as males, and presents earlier in life than other ceruminous gland neoplasms.[19] Histologic features which correlate with worse prognosis include perineural or bone invasion, solid pattern, involvement of the parotid gland, duration of symptoms for greater than 2 years and positive resection margins.[19] Regional lymph node and distant metastases are not uncommon, but of all distant sites, the lungs are the most common.[20,21] Treatment is a lateral temporal bone resection and superficial parotidectomy. A selective neck dissection is indicated for imaging consistent with regional lymphadenopathy. Adjuvant radiation is recommended for close or positive margins, perineural or lymphovascular invasion, bone invasion, solid pattern histology, or lymph node involvement. In one series of 43 patients, the 5-year survival rates for patients with clear surgical margins was 89% and for patients with positive margins was 54%. The 5-year survival rate for patients who received radiation was 62% and those who did not was 86%.[22] Over-all survival is estimated to be approximately 75%.[23]

Ceruminous gland adenocarcinoma not-otherwise-specified

Ceruminous adenocarcinoma is nearly identical to ceruminous adenoma. Microscopic examination will show irregular clusters, nests and sheets of atypical diffusively invasive epithelial cells.[13] Tumors can be classified as high-grade and low-grade tumors depending on the extent of glandular differentiation, but no specific histologic feature has been shown to correlate with patient outcomes.

Ceruminous adenocarcinoma appears to be more common in males and presents most commonly in the 6th to 7th decades of life. Treatment includes complete surgical resection, but it is unknown whether adjuvant radiation improves overall or disease-free survival.[24] Recurrence and metastasis occur frequently despite adequate surgical resection with negative margins.[25] Over-all survival is estimated to be approximately 50%.[23]

Ceruminous mucoepidermoid carcinoma

Ceruminous mucoepidermoid carcinoma of the EAC is extremely rare with only case reports documented in the literature.[26–32] Histologically, it is identical to its salivary gland counterpart. Tumors can be low, intermediate, or high-grade depending on the growth pattern; infiltrative tumors with lymphovascular or perineural invasion, tumor necrosis, high mitotic rate, and cellular pleomorphism all indicate higher grades.

Complete surgical resection is recommended. Robust quantitative survival data is lacking given the rarity of the disease.[23]

Cutaneous

Benign

Squamous papilloma. Squamous papilloma is a benign lesion rarely found in the EAC thought to be caused by the human papilloma virus type 6 and 11.[33,34] The route of transmission is unknown.[34–36] Tumors are fungiform or polypoid with variably sized bases and comprised of well-differentiated stratified squamous epithelium arranged in stalks with a central fibrous core.[33,34] Complete surgical resection is recommended.[37]

Pilomatrixoma. Pilomatrixoma, previously described as calcifying epithelioma of Malherbe, is a benign cutaneous neoplasm arising from primitive hair matrix cells.[38,39] Occurring in the membranous canal, they are solitary firm, cystic, and well-circumscribed. They consist of basaloid cells intermixed with "ghost cells" that have distinct borders but a central unstained area.[40] The majority of diagnoses occur in pediatric patients. Treatment is complete excision.

Malignant

The most common cause of malignancy in the EAC is from extension from the pinna, followed by primary squamous cell carcinoma, basal cell carcinoma, melanoma and Merkel cell carcinoma. Patients can present with symptoms of chronic otitis externa, leading to delays in diagnosis. A high degree of suspicion is warranted, and biopsy should be considered for patients with unresolving symptoms.

Squamous cell carcinoma

Squamous cell carcinoma (SCC) on the helix arises secondary to actinic exposure. SCC arising from the EAC is thought to be related to chronic inflammatory states.[41] Tumors are friable or ulcerated scaly, irregular, and raised. They are characterized by pleomorphic polygonal cells with eosinophilic cytoplasm and intercellular bridging.[42] Tumors are locally invasive and can spread through the cartilaginous canal into the parotid gland and infratemporal fossa, into the postauricular sulcus, through the tympanic membrane and into the middle ear, mastoid, inner ear, and jugular foramen.

The mean age at presentation of lesions on the pinna is the 6th decade of life and for primary EAC lesions, the 5th decade of life. Chronic bloody otorrhea, deep otalgia, facial palsy or sensorineural hearing loss should raise suspicion for invasive malignancy. A timely biopsy followed by a CT to assess for bony invasion and MRI to evaluate for the extent of soft tissue involvement, depth of invasion and perineural invasion are warranted. Regional metastases are common for advanced tumors so regional or full-body imaging are usually performed.

There is no universally accepted staging system for SCC of the ear and temporal bone, however the modified University of Pittsburgh staging system is the most used.[43] In general, tumors limited to the EAC (T1 and T2) have a better prognosis than tumors with the involvement of the middle ear, mastoid, or facial nerve (T3 and T4). Surgery is the standard of care and should involve a lateral temporal bone resection, subtotal temporal bone resection or total temporal bone dissection depending on disease extent. Complete excision with adequate margins is favored, and there is no literature supporting the use of en bloc versus piecemeal resection for either subtotal or total temporal bone resection. Sleeve resections have fallen out of favor because of a high associated recurrence rate.[43] Direct tumor involvement of the parotid gland necessitates a parotidectomy but both elective parotidectomy and neck dissection remain controversial.[43] Adjuvant radiation is recommended for positive margins, perineural invasion, bone invasion and lymph node involvement. Chemotherapy and immunotherapy are both emerging as potential alternatives to surgery followed by adjuvant radiation, but neither are widely utilized yet.[43] The reported 5-year disease free survival rates for combined T1 and T2 tumors and combined T3 and T4 tumor range from 67% to 100% and 41% to 59%, respectively.

Basal cell carcinoma

Basal cell carcinoma (BCC) is the second most common EAC malignancy but accounts for less than 30% of tumors in most series.[44] Actinic exposure is thought to be the primary etiology. Lesions are typically well-circumscribed, displaying a nodular irregularity with rolled edges and a central crusting ulcer but can extend subcutaneously, lacking well-defined margins. Tumors display palisading basaloid cells marginally with central necrosis and ulceration. Histologic subtypes include nodular, sclerosing, morpheaform, superficial spreading, and infiltrative, but tumors can display a mix of subtypes. Most of the BCC of the ear are of the nodular and invasive subtype, but up to 25% might be of morpheaform or sclerosing subtypes.[44] Morpheaform lesions have a propensity for deeper infiltration.

Patients often present in the 6th decade of life with symptoms related to EAC occlusion, but up to one-third might be asymptomatic.[44] Males are affected more commonly than females.[44] Biopsy is required to obtain a diagnosis, and both CT and MRI are used to assess for bony invasion and depth and spread of soft tissue invasion (**Fig. 2**). Though the modified Pittsburgh staging system is commonly used to direct treatment, it appears that BCC overall portends a better prognosis than that of SCC. Surgical resection is the standard of treatment with the choice of limited resection with skin graft, lateral temporal bone resection or composite resection with neck dissection be made based on tumor size and surrounding soft tissue involvement (see **Fig. 2**).[44] Adjuvant radiation should be considered for perineural invasion. The 5-year

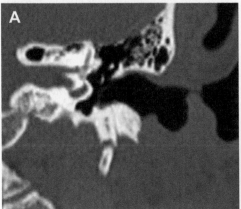
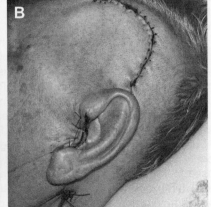

Fig. 2. Preoperative CT temporal bone in the coronal plane (*A*), demonstrating left superior bony external auditory canal soft tissue thickening in a patient diagnosed with primary basal cell carcinoma of the external auditory canal. She underwent a left lateral temporal bone resection, external auditory canal closure and temporalis rotational flap (*B*).

reported disease-free survival is approximately 80%, and the 5-year overall survival is estimated at 78%.[44]

Melanoma

Malignant melanoma arises from melanocytes, derivatives of neural crest cells. Melanomas arising primarily from the EAC make up approximately 5% of primary EAC malignancies.[45] Tumors can be pigmented with changes in color or size or ulceration (**Fig. 3**). Each of five subtypes - superficial spreading, nodular, lentigo, desmoplastic and mucosal – has variable gross and histologic appearances as well as behavior. Superficial spreading is the most common and nodular is the most aggressive. Lentigo maligna has variable pigmentation and desmoplastic may be amelanotic. Tumors are comprised of atypical melanocytes and stain positive for HMB-45, Melan-A, S-100 protein, and vimentin.[45]

Patients often present in the 5th decade of life.[46] The incidence is higher among males than females. Sun exposure is a known risk factor, but there might also be a genetic predisposition.[47] Excisional biopsy of any suspicious lesion should be undertaken. Complete surgical resection is recommended with appropriate margins. Frozen section pathology cannot reliably detect tumor free margins. Primary melanomas might have a propensity for higher stage at diagnosis than melanomas extending from the auricle. En bloc lateral temporal bone resection is recommended.[46] Additionally, current guidelines recommend consideration of a sentinel lymph node biopsy for lesions that are 0.8 mm thick with adverse features and strongly recommend performance of sentinel lymph node biopsy (SLNB) for all lesions greater than 1.0 mm (T2a).[48] Advanced melanoma of the EAC is often treated with adjuvant radiation with improved locoregional control.[49]

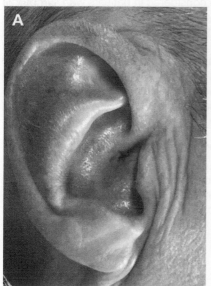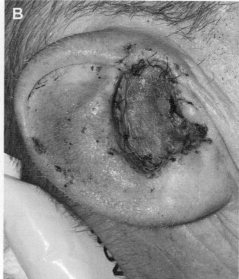

Fig. 3. Clinical photograph of a patient presenting with a discolored, raised lesion centered at the right helical root with extension from the concha cavum toward the meatus (*A*), consistent with malignant melanoma from a dermatologic shave biopsy. He underwent a wide local excision with 1 cm margins involving the meatus and was reconstructed with a split thickness skin graft (*B*).

Several immunotherapeutic agents have been approved for use as well. Distant recurrence is common and disease-free and overall survival outcomes at 1 year are dismal.[46]

Merkel cell carcinoma

Merkel cell carcinoma (MCC) is a rare, aggressive cutaneous neuroendocrine carcinoma.[50] Tumors appear as solitary cutaneous or subcutaneous nodules. Histologically, tumors are comprised of cords, strands or clusters of small, large or intermediate cell sizes, with variably distinct borders, high nucleus to cytoplasmic ratio, salt and pepper appearing nuclei with a small nucleolus. Immunohistochemical staining will differentiate these tumors from other cutaneous malignancies.[50] Risk factors include sun exposure, immunocompromised states or exposure to the polyomavirus.[51,52]

The mean age at presentation is in the 7th decade and males are affected more than females.[53] In addition to developing a rapidly growing, painless nodule of varying hues, approximately 30% of patients will present with regional metastasis.[53] Prompt biopsy and imaging are necessary. Tumor size, infiltrative pattern, thickness and lymphovascular invasion, as well as the presence of regional and distant metastasis are associated with poor prognosis. Recommended treatment includes a wide local excision with 1 to 2 cm margins along with an SLNB or therapeutic neck dissection, followed by adjuvant radiation.[54–57] Local recurrence rates have been reported to be between 40% and 50%.[57,58] Immunotherapy is emerging as a durable option for recurrent and metastatic disease.[57] The estimated 5-year overall survival rates for MCC of all sites is 50% for local disease, 36% for regional metastasis and 14% for distant metastasis.[59]

Metastatic

Metastatic EAC lesions are rare but should be considered in patients with symptoms of chronic non-resolving otitis externa and EAC occlusion with a history of both systemic and nonsystemic malignancies. Metastatic EAC lesions have been reported to arise from parotid, colorectal, bronchogenic, esophageal, rectal, and hepatocellular adenocarcinoma, extrapulmonary small cell carcinoma, prostate carcinoma and renal cell carcinoma.[60–69] Metastatic lesions, most commonly from the breast, lung and prostate, to other regions of the temporal bone might also present as EAC lesions.[70] Up to one-third of patients might be asymptomatic, but of those who are symptomatic, hearing loss, facial paresis and otalgia are the most common symptoms.[70]

Rare neoplasms and those with secondary involvement of the external auditory canal

Primary neoplasms of the middle ear, mastoid, and jugular foramen can present initially as EAC lesions. These include paraganglioma, sarcoma, schwannoma, hemangioma, Langerhans cell histiocytosis, lymphoma, extramedullary plasmacytoma, leukemia, and solitary fibrous tumor. Clinical presentation varies by tumor cell type and extent of disease at the primary site.

SUMMARY

Primary EAC neoplasms include benign and malignant lesions of bony, glandular or cutaneous origin. Benign bony lesions are often asymptomatic, diagnosed incidentally and might not require intervention. Both malignant and benign neoplasms of cutaneous and glandular origin can present with symptoms of chronic otitis externa, leading to delays in diagnosis. Prompt biopsy of soft tissue nodules or lesions associated with non-resolving otitis externa are warranted. Because of the thin EAC skin, even early-stage malignant neoplasms require aggressive surgical treatment. Metastatic neoplasms and lesions arising from other regions of the temporal bone can present in the EAC as well. Therefore, in addition to prompt biopsy, local and regional imaging is helpful to understand disease extent and origin.

CLINICS CARE POINTS

- Osteoma and exostoses do not warrant intervention unless leading to canal obstruction and conductive hearing loss.
- Wide local excision with canalplasty is acceptable management for symptomatic benign cutaneous and glandular neoplasms.
- Cutaneous malignancy should be considered for patients with unresolving otitis externa or non-healing ulcerative or friable lesions.
- Sleeve resection of the EAC skin has a limited role in the management of cutaneous EAC malignancies.

DISCLOSURE

The author has no financial disclosures.

REFERENCES

1. Sandison A. Update from the 5th Edition of the World Health Organization Classification of Head and Neck Tumours: Tumours of the Ear. Head Neck Pathol 2022;16(1):76–86.
2. Swisher AR, Singh P, Debbaneh P, et al. Complication Rates in Osteotome and Drill Techniques in External Auditory Canal Exostoses: A Systematic Review and Meta-Analysis. Ann Otol Rhinol Laryngol 2023. https://doi.org/10.1177/000348942211478804. 34894221147804.
3. Grinblat G, Prasad SC, Piras G, et al. Outcomes of Drill Canalplasty in Exostoses and Osteoma: Analysis of 256 Cases and Literature Review. Otol Neurotol 2016; 37(10):1565–72.
4. Magliulo G, Bertin S. Adenoma of the ceruminous gland. Otolaryngol Head Neck Surg 2010;143(3):459–60.
5. Giuseppe M, Serena B, Sandro B, et al. Adenoma of the ceruminous gland (cerumi- noma). Otol Neurotol 2011;32(2):e14–5.
6. Markou K, Karasmanis I, Vlachtsis K, et al. Primary pleomorphic adenoma of the external ear canal. Report of a case and literature review. Am J Otolaryngol 2008; 29(2):142–6.
7. Thompson LD, Nelson BL, Barnes EL. Ceruminous adenomas: a clinicopathologic study of 41 cases with a review of the literature. Am J Surg Pathol 2004; 28(3):308–18.
8. Arechvo A, Balseris S, Neverauskiene L, et al. Syringocystadenoma papilliferum of the bony external auditory canal: a rare tumor in a rare location. Case Rep Otolaryngol 2013;2013:541679.
9. Bruschini L, Ciabotti A, De Vito A, et al. Syringocystadenoma papilliferum of the external audi- tory canal. Am J Case Rep 2017;18:520–4.

10. Lee CK, Jang KT, Cho YS. Tubular apocrine adenoma with syrin- gocystadenoma papilliferum arising from the external auditory canal. J Laryngol Otol 2005; 119(12):1004–6.

11. Su TC, Shen KH, Wang HK, et al. Lipomatous apocrine adenoma with syringocystadenoma papilliferum arising from the external auditory canal. Head Neck Oncol 2011;3:36.

12. Dehner LP, Chen KT. Primary tumors of the external and middle ear. Benign and malignant glandular neoplasms. Arch Otolaryn- gol. 1980;106(1):13–9.

13. Nagarajan P. Ceruminous Neoplasms of the Ear. Head Neck Pathol 2018;12(3): 350–61.

14. Perzin KH, Gullane P, Conley J. Adenoid cystic carcinoma involving the external auditory canal. A clinicopathologic study of 16 cases. Cancer 1982;50(12): 2873–83.

15. van Weert S, van der Waal I, Witte BI, et al. Histopathological grading of adenoid cystic carcinoma of the head and neck: analysis of currently used grading systems and proposal for a simplified grading scheme. Oral Oncol 2015;51(1):71–6.

16. Fujii K, Murase T, Beppu S, et al. MYB, MYBL1, MYBL2 and NFIB gene alterations and MYC overexpression in salivary gland adenoid cystic carcinoma. His- topathology. 2017;71(5):823–34.

17. Mitani Y, Liu B, Rao PH, et al. Novel MYBL1 gene rearrangements with recurrent MYBL1- NFIB fusions in salivary adenoid cystic carcinomas lacking t(6;9) translocations. Clin Cancer Res 2016;22(3):725–33.

18. Park S, Vora M, van Zante A, et al. Clinicopathologic implications of Myb and Beta-catenin expression in adenoid cystic carcinoma. J Otolaryngol Head Neck Surg 2020;49(1):48.

19. Dong F, Gidley PW, Ho T, et al. Adenoid cystic carcinoma of the external auditory canal. Laryngoscope 2008;118(9):1591–6.

20. Mills RG, Douglas-Jones T, Williams RG. 'Ceruminoma'–a defunct diagnosis. J Laryngol Otol 1995;109(3):180–8.

21. Pulec JL, Parkhill EM, Devine KD. Adenoid cystic carcinoma (cylindroma) of the external auditory canal. Trans Am Acad Ophthalmol Otolaryngol 1963;67:673–94.

22. Gu FM, Chi FL, Dai CF, et al. Surgical outcomes of 43 cases with adenoid cystic carcinoma of the external auditory canal. Am J Otolaryngol 2013;34(5):394–8.

23. Wanner B, Rismiller K, Carr DR. Treatment and survival outcomes of ceruminous carcinomas of the external auditory canal: a SEER database analysis and literature review. Arch Dermatol Res 2022;314(6):583–91.

24. Ruhl DS, Tolisano AM, Swiss TP, et al. Ceruminous adenocarcinoma: An analysis of the Surveillance Epidemiology and End Results (SEER) database. Am J Otolaryngol 2016;37(2):70–3.

25. Jan JC, Wang CP, Kwan PC, et al. Ceruminous adeno- carcinoma with extensive parotid, cervical, and distant metastases: case report and review of literature. Arch Otolaryngol Head Neck Surg 2008;134(6):663–6.

26. Crain N, Nelson BL, Barnes EL, et al. Ceruminous gland carcinomas: a clinicopathologic and immunophenotypic study of 17 cases. Head Neck Pathol 2009; 3(1):1–17.

27. Pulec JL. Glandular tumors of the external auditory canal. Laryngoscope 1977; 87(10 Pt 1):1601–12.

28. Mourad WF, Hu KS, Shourbaji RA, et al. Trimodality approach for ceruminous mucoepidermoid carcinoma of the exter- nal auditory canal. J Laryngol Otol 2013; 127(2):2036.

29. Bared A, Dave SP, Garcia M, et al. Mucoepidermoid car- cinoma of the external auditory canal (EAC). Acta Otolaryngol 2007;127(3):280–4.
30. Chung JH, Lee SH, Park CW, et al. Mucoepidermoid carcinoma in the external auditory canal: a case report. Cancer Res Treat 2012;44(4):275–8.
31. Magliulo G, Ciniglio Appiani M. Mucoepidermoid carcinoma of the external auditory canal. Otolaryngol Head Neck Surg 2010;142(4):624–5.
32. Magliulo G, Ciniglio Appiani M, Colicchio MG, et al. Mucoepidermoid carcinoma of the external auditory canal. Otol Neurotol 2012;33(3):e21–2.
33. Wang S, Yee H, Wen HY, et al. Papillomas of the external ear canal: Report of ten cases in Chinese patients with HPV in situ hybridization. Head Neck Pathol 2009; 3:207–11.
34. Xia MY, Zhu WY, Lu JY, et al. Ultrastructure and human papillomavirus DNA in papillomatosis of external auditory canal. Int J Dermatol 1996;35:337–9.
35. Welsh RL, Gluckman JL. Dissemination of squamous papilloma by surgical manipulation: a case report. Laryngoscope 1984;94(12 pt 1):1568–70.
36. Chang NC, Chien CY, Wu CC, et al. Squamous papilloma in the external auditory canal: A common lesion in an uncommon site. World J Clin Cases 2013;1:92–5.
37. McClellan JH, Ewing E, Gupta S. Squamous papilloma of the external auditory canal. Otol Neurotol 2018;39(5):e413–5.
38. Malherbe A, Chemantais J. Note sur l'epitheliome calcine des glandes sebacees. Pregr Med Paris 1880;8:826–8.
39. Forbes R, Holwig EB. Pilomatrixoma (calcifying epithelioma). Arch Dermatol 1961;83:606–18.
40. Vinayak BC, Cox GJ, Ashton-Key M. Pilomatrixoma of the external auditory meatus. J Laryngol Otol 1993;107(4):333–4.
41. Gaudet JE, Walvekar RR, Arriaga MA, et al. Applicability of the Pittsburgh staging system for advanced cutaneous malignancy of the temporal bone. Skull Base 2010;20:409–14.
42. Allanson BM, Low TH, Clark JR, et al. Squamous Cell Carcinoma of the External Auditory Canal and Temporal Bone: An Update. Head Neck Pathol 2018;12(3): 407–18.
43. Lovin BD, Gidley PW. Squamous cell carcinoma of the temporal bone: A current review. Laryngoscope Investig Otolaryngol 2019;4(6):684–92.
44. Breen JT, Roberts DB, Gidley PW. Basal cell carcinoma of the temporal bone and external auditory canal. Laryngoscope 2018;128(6):1425–30.
45. Langman AW, Yarington CT, Patterson SD. Malignant melanoma of the external auditory canal. Otolaryngol Head Neck Surg 1996;114:645–8.
46. Appelbaum EN, Gross ND, Diab A, et al. Melanoma of the External Auditory Canal: A Review of Seven Cases at a Tertiary Care Referral Center. Laryngoscope 2021;131(1):165–72.
47. Oba J, Woodman SE. The genetic and epigenetic basis of distinct melanoma types. J Dermatol 2021;48(7):925–39.
48. NCCN guidelines for cutaneous melanoma. Plymouth Meeting, PA: National Comprehensive Cancer Network; 2019.
49. Agrawal S, Kane JM, Guadagnolo BA, et al. The benefits of adjuvant radiation therapy after therapeutic lymphadenectomy for clinically advanced, high-risk, lymph node-metastatic melanoma. Cancer 2009;115:5836–44.
50. Rindi G, Mete O, Uccella S, et al. Overview of the 2022 WHO Classification of Neuroendocrine Neoplasms. Endocr Pathol 2022;33(1):115–54.
51. Feng H, Shuda M, Chang Y, et al. Clonal Integration of a Polyomavirus in Human Merkel Cell Carcinoma. Science 2008;319:1096–100.

52. Wong SQ, Waldeck K, Vergara IA, et al. UV-Associated Mutations Underlie the Etiology of MCV-Negative Merkel Cell Carcinomas. Cancer Res 2015;75: 5228–34.
53. Alves AS, Scampa M, Martineau J, et al. Merkel Cell Carcinoma of the External Ear: Population-Based Analysis and Survival Outcomes. Cancers 2022;14(22): 5653.
54. Maloney N, Nguyen K, So N, et al. Risk factors for and prognostic impact of positive surgical margins after excision of Merkel cell carcinoma. J Am Acad Dermatol 2021;87:444–6.
55. Tai PA. Practical Update of Surgical Management of Merkel Cell Carcinoma of the Skin. ISRN Surg 2013;2013:850797.
56. Jouary T, Leyral C, Dreno B, et al. Adjuvant prophylactic regional radiotherapy versus observation in stage I Merkel cell carcinoma: A multicentric prospective randomized study. Ann Oncol 2011;23:1074–80.
57. Zaggana E, Konstantinou MP, Krasagakis GH, et al. Merkel Cell Carcinoma-Update on Diagnosis, Management and Future Perspectives. Cancers 2022; 15(1):103.
58. Poulsen M. Merkel-cell carcinoma of the skin. Lancet Oncol 2004;5(10):593–9.
59. Harms KL, Healy MA, Nghiem P, et al. Analysis of Prognostic Factors from 9387 Merkel Cell Carcinoma Cases Forms the Basis for the New 8th Edition AJCC Staging System. Ann Surg Oncol 2016;23:3564–71.
60. Lee DH, Kim JH, Chung IJ, et al. Metastasis of parotid adenocarcinoma to the external auditory canal. Ear Nose Throat J 2022. 1455613221086033.
61. James A, Karandikar S, Baijal S. External auditory canal lesion: colorectal metastatic adenocarcinoma. BMJ Case Rep 2018;2018. bcr2018224876.
62. Vasileiadis I, Kapetanakis S, Vasileiadis D, et al. External auditory canal mass as the first manifestation of a bronchogenic carcinoma: report of a rare case. Ann Otol Rhinol Laryngol 2013;122(6):378–81.
63. Rudman KL, King E, Poetker DM. Extrapulmonary small cell carcinoma metastasis to the external auditory canal with facial nerve paralysis. Am J Otolaryngol 2011;32(4):343–5.
64. Lollar KW, Parker CA, Liess BD, et al. Metastatic esophageal adenocarcinoma presenting as an external auditory canal mass. Otolaryngol Head Neck Surg 2010;142(2):298–9.
65. Carr S, Anderson C. Metastatic rectal adenocarcinoma in the external auditory canal. J Laryngol Otol 2009;123(3):363–4.
66. Yasumatsu R, Okura K, Sakiyama Y, et al. Metastatic hepatocellular carcinoma of the external auditory canal. World J Gastroenterol 2007;13(47):6436–8.
67. Shrivastava V, Christensen R, Poggi MM. Prostate cancer metastatic to the external auditory canals. Clin Genitourin Cancer 2007;5(5):341–3.
68. Michaelson PG, Lowry TR. Metastatic renal cell carcinoma presenting in the external auditory canal. Otolaryngol Head Neck Surg 2005;133(6):979–80.
69. Goldman NC, Hutchison RE, Goldman MS. Metastatic renal cell carcinoma of the external auditory canal. Otolaryngol Head Neck Surg 1992;106(4):410–1.
70. Jones AJ, Tucker BJ, Novinger LJ, et al. Metastatic Disease of the Temporal Bone: A Contemporary Review. Laryngoscope 2021;131(5):1101–9.

Radiotherapy-induced Pathology of the Ear

Kaitlyn A. Brooks, MD[a], Jennifer H. Gross, MD[a],*

KEYWORDS

- Radiotherapy • External ear • External auditory canal
- Soft tissue pathologic condition • Otitis externa • Radiation-induced dermatitis

KEY POINTS

- Acute radiotherapy (RT)-induced soft tissue changes include erythema and dry desquamation, which may be followed by moist desquamation and epithelial ulceration. Acute changes usually resolve 4 to 6 weeks after RT conclusion.
- Chronic RT-induced soft tissue change includes epithelial atrophy, subcutaneous fibrosis, and poor healing capabilities.
- Patients with otitis externa after or during radiation should receive topical antimicrobial steroidal treatment and may benefit from systemic treatment and external ear cleaning.
- Topical steroid therapy has promising early data for treatment of radiation dermatitis, but this has not been studied in the external auditory canal.

BACKGROUND

Radiotherapy (RT) has become a mainstay for definitive or adjuvant therapy for head and neck cancer. Recent technological advances, such as photon intensity modulated radiation therapy (IMRT) and intensity modulated proton therapy (IMPT), have improved targeting from conventional RT. Conformal RT, introduced in the 1990s, provided a novel method for matching high RT doses with irregular tumor shapes and decreased long-term RT-related side effects when compared with conventional RT.[1] IMRT, a subset of conformal RT, uses radiation beams of nonuniform intensity to treat the 3-dimensional tumor shape with higher precision.[2] IMPT has a unique depth-dose that stops proton energy at a set distance, meaning that tissues do not receive radiation upon exit of the beam. Although multiple studies suggest that IMPT may be associated with decreased radiation toxicity and side effects,[3,4] this question will be answered with prospective randomized trials that are currently underway.

---

[a] Department of Otolaryngology–Head and Neck Surgery, Emory University, Atlanta, GA 30308, USA
* Corresponding author. Department of Otolaryngology, Emory University Hospital Midtown, 550 Peachtree Street NE, 11th Floor, Atlanta, GA 30308.
E-mail address: Jennifer.helen.gross@emory.edu

Otolaryngol Clin N Am 56 (2023) 977–985
https://doi.org/10.1016/j.otc.2023.05.013
0030-6665/23/© 2023 Elsevier Inc. All rights reserved.

Nondiseased organs in the head and neck, however, still experience collateral radiation toxicity. Berg and Lindgren[5] were the first to explore how radiation changes the external auditory canal (EAC) in 1961, describing an initial epithelial hyperplasia with low-dose RT that transformed into epithelial erosion, ulceration, and suppuration at higher doses. This article focuses on how radiation alters the soft tissue of the external ear, current management strategies to prevent progression, and future directions of treatment.

PATHOGENESIS

RT kills malignant cells by inducing free radicals[6,7] and reactive oxygen species, which cause cellular damage by dismantling DNA and proteins.[6] When skin and subcutaneous tissue are injured, the tissue responds by attempting to heal. Immediate hemostasis, inflammation (days 0–4), proliferation (day 3 to weeks), and remodeling (weeks to years) constitute this multistep, complex process.[6] Although rigorously organized in healthy tissue, postradiation healing is altered because of broad exposure, repeated insult, and cyclic reactivation of the inflammatory cascade. Cytokines attract neutrophils, monocytes, and lymphocytes.[8] Monocytes transform into macrophages as they enter the irradiated soft tissue and stimulate fibroblast migration and maturation. Macrophages, fibroblasts, and epithelial cells secrete transforming growth factor-beta, which activates a fibrotic pathway that persists long after radiation concludes.[8–11] Soft tissue fibrosis ultimately leads to decreased tissue perfusion[12] and lymphovascular drainage, resulting in frail tissue that exhibits poor healing capabilities.[13,14]

Skin and soft tissue are especially radiosensitive, which is indicated by the high frequency of adverse skin reactions (>95%) during radiation therapy.[6,15] Radiation-induced dermatitis is a well-known phenomenon,[16,17] and its severity is classified with the National Cancer Institute (NCI) Common Terminology Criteria for Adverse Events (CTCAE) criteria, shown in **Table 1**.[18]

NATURE OF THE PROBLEM

The auricle and the EAC make up the external ear; both structures are lined with keratinized stratified squamous epithelium.[19] The auricle is a soft, fibrocartilaginous structure that transitions into the lateral cartilaginous third of the EAC. The EAC is a skin-lined pouch originating at the auricle and ending at the tympanic membrane, which separates the external ear from the middle ear.[20] The auricle and lateral EAC

Table 1		
National Cancer Institute Common Terminology Criteria for Adverse Events severity grading for radiation-induced dermatitis		
Severity	**Physical Findings**	
Grade 1	Faint erythema with dry desquamation	
Grade 2	Moderate erythema and edema with patchy, moist desquamation, mostly confined to skin creases	
Grade 3	Confluent, widespread moist desquamation, bleeding is common with trauma	
Grade 4	Skin necrosis or full-thickness dermis ulceration, spontaneous bleeding can occur	
Grade 5	Death due to dermatitis	

Data from Ref.[18]

possess thicker epithelium with pilosebaceous units. The medial two-thirds of the EAC spans the junction between the lateral cartilaginous framework and the tympanic bone to the external surface of the tympanic membrane and is covered by a thin epithelium closely adherent to the underlying periosteum of the bony EAC.

RT-induced soft tissue changes happen acutely (≤30 days of initial exposure) and chronically. Common acute changes include erythema, which sets in hours after radiation, and both dry and moist epithelial desquamation, which occur 3 to 4 weeks after initial RT exposure.[21–23] Erythema and dry epithelial desquamation are shown in **Fig. 1**. Initial erythema is similar to a sunburn and consists of hyperemia and inflammation.[16] With moist desquamation, patients begin to experience otorrhea, similar to **Fig. 2**.[23] Secondary epithelial ulceration can be seen 6 weeks into RT[22]; when this happens, the patient may experience significant otalgia and worsening serous otorrhea.[21,24] Most acute soft tissue reactions resolve spontaneously 4 to 6 weeks after the conclusion of RT.[25] **Table 2** shows the different ways acute external ear toxicity severity has been classified by the NCI CTCAE.[18,26]

With disruption of the protective squamous barrier and a proinflammatory environment, otitis externa can develop with worsening edema and purulent otorrhea. Desquamation combined with edema can result in keratinous debris accumulating in the external ear canal, in turn further obstructing evacuation of debris from the canal and sound propagation.[23] Robinson[23] described 4 cases of RT-induced otitis externa in the 1990s, with growth of *Staphylococcus aureus*, coagulase negative *Staphylococcus*, *Diphtheroids*, and *Pseudomonas aeruginosa* isolated from the EAC. Complete resolution of the radiation-induced otitis externa took from 1 to 18 months.[23] More recent data show that chronic otitis externa occurs in 1% to 3% of patients who receive high-dose RT (55–70 Gy) and in 0% of patients who underwent medium-dose RT (40–55 Gy).[27]

Chronic effects of radiation include atrophy of the epidermis, dermis, and pilosebaceous units as shown in **Fig. 3**, resulting in a thinner epithelium, which is inherently more vulnerable to injury and poor wound healing.[6,13,28] After conclusion of RT, atrophy begins after 12 weeks, and subcutaneous fibrosis begins after 6 to 12 months and continues to progress over time.[22,24] Rates of late auricular skin and cartilage necrosis

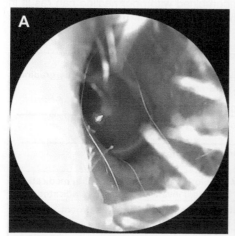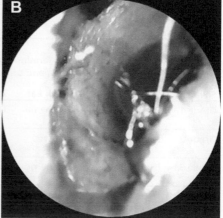

Fig. 1. A 59-year-old woman with salivary duct carcinoma of the right parotid gland who has received 29 Gy proton RT (total planned 63 Gy). (*A*) Nonradiated left EAC. (*B*) Irradiated right ear with faint erythema and dry desquamation, similar to grade 1 external ear toxicity.

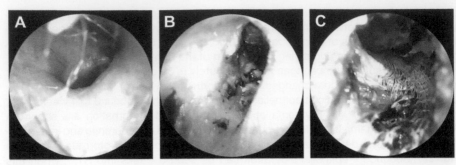

Fig. 2. An 84-year-old man with squamous cell carcinoma of the left parotid gland who has received 40 Gy proton RT (total planned 60 Gy). (*A*) Nonradiated right EAC. (*B*) Irradiated left lateral EAC with bleeding and moist desquamation, which extends medially to the bony EAC as shown in (*C*), similar to grade 3 acute radiation dermatitis and external ear toxicity.

have been historically reported in up to 13% of patients undergoing conventional irradiation of the pinna for superficial cutaneous carcinomas,[25,29,30] but these complications have not been seen with IMRT and IMPT. Canal cholesteatoma[28] and EAC stenosis[27] have also been reported with chronic soft tissue changes. Radiation-induced EAC stenosis has been seen in 8.7% of patients who receive high-dose RT (55–75 Gy) and is higher risk in patients who underwent surgery adjacent to the EAC, such as parotidectomy.[27] Canal cholesteatoma and acquired stenosis will be discussed in detail in separate articles.

PREVENTION

Patients who have their external ear in the radiation field need to be instructed to keep their ears as dry as possible to avoid infection.[23] Before the start of RT, patients should have their ears cleaned and inspected to promote proper ventilation of the EAC. With atrophy of the epithelium, patients should be counseled to avoid blindly placing objects into the EAC, as self-inflicted trauma combined with poor healing can result in worsening pathologic condition.[31] Monthly application of mineral oil has been

Table 2		
National Cancer Institute Common Terminology Criteria for Adverse Events severity grading comparison for external ear in 1999, and otitis externa in 2017		
Severity	**1999 NCI CTCAE External Ear**	**2017 NCI CTCAE Otitis Externa**
Grade 1	External otitis with erythema or dry desquamation	Localized intervention indicated
Grade 2	External otitis with moist desquamation	Oral intervention indicated
Grade 3	External otitis with discharge	IV antibiotic, antifungal, or antiviral medication indicated; invasive intervention indicated
Grade 4	Necrosis of the canal soft tissue or bone	Life-threatening consequences; urgent intervention indicated
Grade 5	N/A	Death

Abbreviation: N/A, not applicable.
Criteria from Ref.[26] and data from Ref.[18]

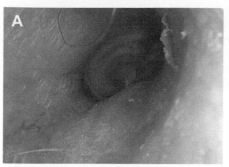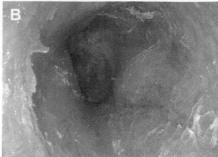

Fig. 3. A 72-year-old man with a history of left nasopharyngeal carcinoma status post definitive chemoradiation (70 Gy). (*A*) Nonradiated right EAC for comparison. (*B*) Irradiated left EAC with thinned epidermis and dry sloughing consistent with chronic radiation change.

suggested as a lubricating agent for the EAC to prevent injury, late epithelial necrosis, and ulceration for patients who have completed radiation.[21,32]

THERAPEUTICS

Management of acute radiation-induced soft tissue EAC disease is not well protocolized and has not been recently studied. Robinson[23] treated 4 cases of RT-induced otitis externa with frequent aural toilet and cleaning, placement of ribbon gauze, and 1% aqueous solution of Gentian Violet in the 1990s. Robinson[23] suggested that excessive topical and oral antibiotics use can prolong RT-induced otitis externa owing to growth of opportunistic organisms, but specific regimens for RT-induced otitis externa have not been described since. Current otitis externa treatment guidelines state that systemic antimicrobial therapy may be beneficial in addition to topical antimicrobial therapy.[33] Leonetti and colleagues[32] stated that topical antibiotic and steroidal drops should be prescribed in cases of skin ulceration to prevent infection and progression to temporal bone osteoradionecrosis. Topical corticosteroids have been used to treat chondritis and external EAC irritation.[25]

Radiation dermatitis, however, has been thoroughly studied. Grade 1 dermatitis (faint erythema and dry desquamation) is managed with routine hygiene and routine daily application of hydrophilic moisturizers.[34] Treatment of grade 2 or 3 dermatitis (moist desquamation) focuses on preventing secondary infection and protecting sloughing skin with dressings. Grade 4 dermatitis is particularly rare; the patient may require discontinuation of radiation and specialized wound care.[34] Patients with symptomatic discomfort and pruritis are treated with topical corticosteroids,[34] and daily application during RT has been shown to decrease rates of wet desquamation.[35,36] A randomized controlled trial[37] was conducted for radiation dermatitis treatment comparing topical steroid with hydrophilic ointment application. When grade 1 dermatitis was observed, the patient experienced pruritis, or when 30 Gy total radiation dose was reached, the intervention arm applied topical difluprednate versus petrolatum to the irradiated skin. The number of patients who suffered from grade 2 radiation dermatitis was similar between the 2 groups, but the number of patients who progressed to grade 3 dermatitis was significantly lower in the topical steroid group.

For late RT-induced complications, randomized controlled trials for patients with breast cancer have demonstrated prevention[38] and even regression[39] of subcutaneous fibrosis with prolonged treatment with pentoxifylline and vitamin E. The dosing recommendations have not been well-defined, but Delanian and colleagues[39] used 800 mg daily of pentoxifylline in combination with 1000 Units per day of vitamin E. Magnusson and colleagues[38] used an incremental dosing increase of pentoxifylline (400 mg daily for 2 weeks, 400 mg twice daily for 2 weeks, and then 400 mg 3 times daily) in combination with 100 mg vitamin E 3 times daily. The most common side effect related to this regimen was nausea, which was attributed to the pentoxifylline. Pentoxifylline and vitamin E have been studied for osteoradionecrosis of the temporal bone and EAC,[40] but not for RT-induced soft tissue EAC disease. Hyperbaric oxygen therapy (HBO) has been used for both osteoradionecrosis of the mandible[41] and of the temporal bone,[42,43] but its effects on EAC RT-induced soft tissue disease are unclear. HBO works by prompting angiogenesis and alteration in fibrous tissue, effectively restoring the organized proliferation and healing of epithelium.[44]

Traditional hearing aids can be troublesome for irradiated patients because of possible EAC irritation, which is posited as a risk for otitis and osteoradionecrosis.[45] Nader and Gidley[46] determined that hearing aid fitting should be done with special care to avoid models that will exert EAC pressure. Patients with head and neck cancer requiring amplification owing to sensorineural hearing loss are typically fitted with behind-the-ear devices with an open-fit dome.[46] Osseointegrated hearing aids are an option for patients with significant otorrhea and soft tissue changes precluding the use of conventional hearing aids.[21,47] The concern of decreased rates of osseointegration, however, is pertinent; implant survival rate is quoted between 83% and 100%.[46]

DISCUSSION

There is a paucity of literature addressing the treatment of RT-induced soft tissue disease of the external ear and the subsequent progression to temporal bone osteoradionecrosis. There is good evidence, however, to support management strategies of RT-induced dermatitis that can be applied to the external ear.[36,37] The varying levels of severity of RT-induced dermatitis (erythema, dry desquamation, or moist desquamation) can be applied to otoscopic examination to determine if topical corticosteroid treatment may be beneficial. However, the EAC is more challenging to visualize for a nonspecialist, and otolaryngologists do not routinely see patients during RT unless their symptoms warrant specialized evaluation.

Routine otologic examination for patients whose radiation field includes the temporal bone may be useful to identify grade 1 dermatitis of the EAC, as these patients may benefit from topical steroid therapy. The current otitis externa guidelines recommend that patients with otitis externa and a history of RT may benefit from systemic treatment in addition to topical antimicrobial agents.[33] Increased attention to external ear soft tissue disease after radiation may decrease the risk of progression to osteoradionecrosis, but interventions that have been applied in the field of radiation oncology for dermatitis and emerging interventions warrant further study.

SUMMARY

Acute RT-induced external ear soft tissue changes typically start early during the radiation course with erythema and dry desquamation and may progress to moist desquamation and epidermal ulceration. Chronic RT-induced changes include epithelial atrophy and subcutaneous fibrosis. After RT, patients should avoid EAC trauma. Interventions for EAC soft tissue pathologic condition include topical steroid treatment for erythema and dry desquamation and topical antibiotic therapy for suppurative otitis externa; topical corticosteroid treatment may prevent worsening of RT-induced soft tissue disease. Interventions for soft tissue radionecrosis involving the EAC warrant further investigation.

CLINICS CARE POINTS

- Acute radiotherapy-induced soft tissue changes include erythema and dry desquamation first, which may be followed by moist desquamation and epithelial ulceration.
- Chronic radiotherapy-induced soft tissue changes include epithelial atrophy, subcutaneous fibrosis, and overall poor wound-healing capabilities.
- Patients with otitis externa after or during radiation should receive topical antimicrobial steroidal treatment and may benefit from systemic treatment.
- Topical steroid therapy is promising for radiation dermatitis management but has not been studied in the external auditory canal.
- Hearing aid fitting and selection for irradiated patients should aim for minimal irritation and applied pressure to the external auditory canal.

DISCLOSURE

The authors testify no financial relationships to disclose or conflicts of interest pertaining to this work.

REFERENCES

1. Dearnaley DP, Khoo VS, Norman AR, et al. Comparison of radiation side-effects of conformal and conventional radiotherapy in prostate cancer: a randomised trial. Lancet 1999;353(9149):267–72.
2. Taylor A, Powell ME. Intensity-modulated radiotherapy–what is it? Cancer Imag 2004;4(2):68–73.
3. Moreno AC, Frank SJ, Garden AS, et al. Intensity modulated proton therapy (IMPT) - The future of IMRT for head and neck cancer. Oral Oncol 2019;88:66–74.
4. Sio TT, Lin HK, Shi Q, et al. Intensity modulated proton therapy versus intensity modulated photon radiation therapy for oropharyngeal cancer: first comparative results of patient-reported outcomes. Int J Radiat Oncol Biol Phys 2016;95(4): 1107–14.
5. Berg NO, Lindgren M. Dose factors and morphology of delayed radiation lesions of the internal and middle ear in rabbits. Acta Radiol 1961;56:305–19.
6. Dormand EL, Banwell PE, Goodacre TE. Radiotherapy and wound healing. Int Wound J 2005;2(2):112–27.
7. Bentzen SM. Preventing or reducing late side effects of radiation therapy: radiobiology meets molecular pathology. Nat Rev Cancer 2006;6(9):702–13.
8. Borrelli MR, Shen AH, Lee GK, et al. Radiation-Induced Skin Fibrosis: Pathogenesis, Current Treatment Options, and Emerging Therapeutics. Ann Plast Surg 2019;83(4S Suppl 1):S59–64.
9. Randall K, Coggle JE. Expression of transforming growth factor-beta 1 in mouse skin during the acute phase of radiation damage. Int J Radiat Biol 1995;68(3):301–9.
10. Vegesna V, McBride WH, Taylor JM, et al. The effect of interleukin-1 beta or transforming growth factor-beta on radiation-impaired murine skin wound healing. J Surg Res 1995;59(6):699–704.

11. Martin M, Lefaix J, Delanian S. TGF-beta1 and radiation fibrosis: a master switch and a specific therapeutic target? Int J Radiat Oncol Biol Phys 2000;47(2):277–90.

12. Rohleder NH, Flensberg S, Bauer F, et al. Can tissue spectrophotometry and laser Doppler flowmetry help to identify patients at risk for wound healing disorders after neck dissection? Oral Surg Oral Med Oral Pathol Oral Radiol 2014; 117(3):302–11.

13. Koerdt S, Rohleder NH, Rommel N, et al. An expression analysis of markers of radiation-induced skin fibrosis and angiogenesis in wound healing disorders of the head and neck. Radiat Oncol 2015;10:202.

14. Wang J, Boerma M, Fu Q, et al. Radiation responses in skin and connective tissues: effect on wound healing and surgical outcome. Hernia 2006;10(6):502–6.

15. Porock D, Nikoletti S, Kristjanson L. Management of radiation skin reactions: literature review and clinical application. Plast Surg Nurs. Winter 1999;19(4):185–92, 223; [quiz: 191-2].

16. Hymes SR, Strom EA, Fife C. Radiation dermatitis: clinical presentation, pathophysiology, and treatment 2006. J Am Acad Dermatol 2006;54(1):28–46.

17. Takagi M, Demizu Y, Hashimoto N, et al. Treatment outcomes of particle radiotherapy using protons or carbon ions as a single-modality therapy for adenoid cystic carcinoma of the head and neck. Radiother Oncol 2014;113(3):364–70.

18. National Cancer Institute: Division of Cancer Treatment and Diagnosis. Common Terminology Criteria for Adverse Events (CTCAE) Version 2. In: Cancer Therapy and Evaluation Program. 1999. Available at: https://ctep.cancer.gov/protocol development/electronic_applications/docs/ctcv20_4-30-992.pdf. Accessed March 6, 2023.

19. Ansari A, Tariq MA, Sadiq NM. Histology, Ear. In: StatPearls. 2023. Available at: https://www.ncbi.nlm.nih.gov/books/NBK545170/. Accessed February 23, 2023.

20. Luong A, Roland PS. Acquired external auditory canal stenosis: assessment and management. Curr Opin Otolaryngol Head Neck Surg 2005;13(5):273–6.

21. Jereczek-Fossa BA, Zarowski A, Milani F, et al. Radiotherapy-induced ear toxicity. Cancer Treat Rev 2003;29(5):417–30.

22. Brown KR, Rzucidlo E. Acute and chronic radiation injury. J Vasc Surg 2011;53(1 Suppl):15S–21S.

23. Robinson AC. Management of radiation-induced otitis externa. J Laryngol Otol 1990;104(6):458–9.

24. Million RR, Parsons JT, Mendenhall WM. Effect of radiation on normal tissues in the head and neck. Bone, cartilage, and soft tissue. Front Radiat Ther Oncol 1989;23:221–37 [discussion: 251-4].

25. Lim JT. Irradiation of the pinna with superficial kilovoltage radiotherapy. Clin Oncol 1992;4(4):236–9.

26. National Cancer Institute: Division of Cancer Treatment and Diagnosis. Common Terminology Criteria for Adverse Events (CTCAE) Version 5. In: Cancer Therapy and Evaluation Program. 2017. Available at: https://ctep.cancer.gov/protocol development/electronic_applications/docs/CTCAE_v5_Quick_Reference_8.5x11. pdf. Accessed March 6, 2023.

27. Carls JL, Mendenhall WM, Morris CG, et al. External auditory canal stenosis after radiation therapy. Laryngoscope 2002;112(11):1975–8.

28. Adler M, Hawke M, Berger G, et al. Radiation effects on the external auditory canal. J Otolaryngol 1985;14(4):226–32.

29. Silva JJ, Tsang RW, Panzarella T, et al. Results of radiotherapy for epithelial skin cancer of the pinna: the Princess Margaret Hospital experience, 1982-1993. Int J Radiat Oncol Biol Phys 2000;47(2):451–9.

30. Hayter CR, Lee KH, Groome PA, et al. Necrosis following radiotherapy for carcinoma of the pinna. Int J Radiat Oncol Biol Phys 1996;36(5):1033–7.
31. Yuhan BT, Nguyen BK, Svider PF, et al. Osteoradionecrosis of the temporal bone: an evidence-based approach. Otol Neurotol 2018;39(9):1172–83.
32. Leonetti JP, Origitano T, Anderson D, et al. Intracranial complications of temporal bone osteoradionecrosis. Am J Otol 1997;18(2):223–8 [discussion: 228-9].
33. Rosenfeld RM, Schwartz SR, Cannon CR, et al. Clinical practice guideline: acute otitis externa. Otolaryngol Head Neck Surg 2014;150(1 Suppl):S1–24.
34. Wong RK, Bensadoun RJ, Boers-Doets CB, et al. Clinical practice guidelines for the prevention and treatment of acute and late radiation reactions from the MASCC skin toxicity study group. Support Care Cancer 2013;21(10):2933–48.
35. Haruna F, Lipsett A, Marignol L. Topical management of acute radiation dermatitis in breast cancer patients: a systematic review and meta-analysis. Anticancer Res 2017;37(10):5343–53.
36. Ho AY, Olm-Shipman M, Zhang Z, et al. A randomized trial of mometasone furoate 0.1% to reduce high-grade acute radiation dermatitis in breast cancer patients receiving postmastectomy radiation. Int J Radiat Oncol Biol Phys 2018;101(2): 325–33.
37. Yokota T, Zenda S, Ota I, et al. Phase 3 randomized trial of topical steroid versus placebo for prevention of radiation dermatitis in patients with head and neck cancer receiving chemoradiation. Int J Radiat Oncol Biol Phys 2021;111(3):794–803.
38. Magnusson M, Hoglund P, Johansson K, et al. Pentoxifylline and vitamin E treatment for prevention of radiation-induced side-effects in women with breast cancer: a phase two, double-blind, placebo-controlled randomised clinical trial (Ptx-5). Eur J Cancer 2009;45(11):2488–95.
39. Delanian S, Porcher R, Balla-Mekias S, et al. Randomized, placebo-controlled trial of combined pentoxifylline and tocopherol for regression of superficial radiation-induced fibrosis. J Clin Oncol 2003;21(13):2545–50.
40. Lovin BD, Choi JS, Lindquist NR, et al. Pentoxifylline and tocopherol in the management of temporal bone osteoradionecrosis: a case series. Otol Neurotol 2020; 41(10):1438–46.
41. Forner LE, Dieleman FJ, Shaw RJ, et al. Hyperbaric oxygen treatment of mandibular osteoradionecrosis: combined data from the two randomized clinical trials DAHANCA-21 and NWHHT2009-1. Radiother Oncol 2022;166:137–44.
42. Sharon JD, Khwaja SS, Drescher A, et al. Osteoradionecrosis of the temporal bone: a case series. Otol Neurotol 2014;35(7):1207–17.
43. Metselaar M, Dumans AG, van der Huls MP, et al. Osteoradionecrosis of tympanic bone: reconstruction of outer ear canal with pedicled skin flap, combined with hyperbaric oxygen therapy, in five patients. J Laryngol Otol 2009;123(10): 1114–9.
44. Ashamalla HL, Thom SR, Goldwein JW. Hyperbaric oxygen therapy for the treatment of radiation-induced sequelae in children. The University of Pennsylvania experience. Cancer 1996;77(11):2407–12.
45. Lambert EM, Gunn GB, Gidley PW. Effects of radiation on the temporal bone in patients with head and neck cancer. Head Neck 2016;38(9):1428–35.
46. Nader ME, Gidley PW. Challenges of Hearing rehabilitation after radiation and chemotherapy. J Neurol Surg B Skull Base 2019;80(2):214–24.
47. Soo G, Tong MC, Tsang WS, et al. The BAHA hearing system for hearing-impaired postirradiated nasopharyngeal cancer patients: a new indication. Otol Neurotol 2009;30(4):496–501.

Skull Base Osteomyelitis
Historical Perspective, Diagnosis and Management Update

Mickie Hamiter, MD[a], Valerianna Amorosa, MD[b],
Katherine Belden, MD[c], Paul W. Gidley, MD, FACS[d],
Suyash Mohan, MD[e], Brian Perry, MD[f], Ana H. Kim, MD[a,*]

KEYWORDS

- Skull base osteomyelitis (SBO) • Malignant otitis externa (MOE) • Diabetes mellitus

KEY POINTS

- The hallmark presenting symptom of SBO is otalgia, typically described as a persistent and severe deep pain with nocturnal worsening.
- SBO is a chronic bone infection with high morbidity and mortality.
- Appropriate duration of medical treatment is crucial to avoid incomplete treatment that results in relapse and complications.

HISTORICAL PERSPECTIVE AND NOMENCLATURE

The clinical entity which is known to cause severe otalgia and otorrhea, with potential progression to cranial nerve palsies, intracranial complications, and ultimately death, in an elderly diabetic or immunocompromised population has been given a variety of names over the past 150 years, including temporal bone osteomyelitis,[1] diabetic ear,[2] necrotizing otitis externa,[3] malignant external otitis,[4] and finally skull base osteomyelitis.[5] Each "name" has merit and shortcomings. "Diabetic ear" does not allow for other

[a] Department of Otolaryngology, Columbia University Irving Medical Center, New York, NY, USA; [b] Module E, First floor, Corporal Michael J. Crescenz VA Medical Center, University and Woodlawn Avenue, Philadelphia, PA 19104, USA; [c] Division of Infectious Diseases, Thomas Jefferson University Hospital, 1101 Market Street, Suite 2720, Philadelphia, PA 19107, USA; [d] Department of Head and Neck Surgery, UT MD Anderson Cancer Center, 1515 Holcombe Boulevard, Unit 1445, Houston, TX 77030, USA; [e] Department of Radiology, 219 Dulles Building, Hospital of the University of Pennsylvania, 3400 Spruce Street, Philadelphia, PA 19004, USA; [f] Department of OTO-HNS, UT Health San Antonio, Joe R. and Teresa Lozano Long School of Medicine, 7703 Floyd Curl Drive, MC 7777, San Antonio, TX 78229-3900, USA
* Corresponding author. Department of Otolaryngology, Columbia University Medical Center, 180 Fort Washington, Harkness Pavilion 8-864, New York, NY 10032
E-mail address: ahk2166@cumc.columbia.edu

Otolaryngol Clin N Am 56 (2023) 987–1001
https://doi.org/10.1016/j.otc.2023.06.004
0030-6665/23/© 2023 Elsevier Inc. All rights reserved.

oto.theclinics.com

causes of an immunocompromised state that can also lead to a severe otologic infection, including children and adults receiving chemotherapy, individuals with HIV, those on immunosuppressives, and the elderly. Chandler 1968 coined the term malignant external otitis to describe "a severe infection which tends to occur in elderly patients with diabetes ... which may be responsible for multiple cranial nerve palsies, meningitis and death."[4] Necrotizing otitis externa (external otitis) was first coined by Kohut 1979 to confirm that the disease is not "malignant,"[6] It emphasizes the nature of the disease as a progressive cellulitis of the ear and skull base. Finally, skull base osteomyelitis by Nadol 1980 has been employed to describe the observed pathology, including active osteomyelitis along the sigmoid sulcus, posterior fossa surface of the temporal bone, and petrous apex.[5] As skull base osteomyelitis (SBO) most accurately describes this disease process, without the potential confusion with a "cancerous lesion," it will be used exclusively in this article with the exception of describing results from historical literature.

Toulmouche 1838 was the first to describe this ailment with intracranial complications in "Observations d'Otorrhee Cerebrale; Suivis des Reflexions,"[7] The organism responsible for this life-threatening infection was identified by Zaufal 1873 and called *Vibrio cyanagenus*; now referred to as *Pseudomonas aeruginosa*.[8] Chambers 1900 reported on 6 cases of severe otologic infections caused by *V cyanagenus*, three of which died of the infection.[9] Wakefield 1904 and Voss 1906 both described intracranial complications and death from pyocyaneus otologic infections.[10,11] The first animal models of otitis externa were reported in 1914 using guinea pig and in 1926 with a mouse model.[12,13] Both animal models demonstrated suppurative labyrinthitis following ear canal inoculation with *V cyanagenus*. The pathologic changes occurring in the temporal bone were likely first described by Brunner in 1942, which he termed "acute, protracted, progressive osteomyelitis." He also reported a characteristic leaping from focus to focus of osteomyelitis, which indicated a hematogenous spread, rather than direct extension through the pneumatized spaces.[1,14] A detailed description of the clinical course of disease with a pathologic correlate was not reported until 1959.[3] These authors chronicled a patient with "severe" diabetes who developed acute otitis externa with Pseudomonas, and despite aggressive medical and multiple radical surgical procedures (including 2 radical mastoidectomies, infratemporal fossa approach for removal of abscess cavity, TMJ and mandible, resection of both internal and external carotid) the patient died 8 months after initial diagnosis. They too demonstrated the spread of disease along vascular channels rather than through the pneumatized spaces of the mastoid and petrous apex, differentiating this disease process from acute or chronic mastoiditis.

Chandler coined the term malignant external otitis when reporting on 13 patients with "a particularly severe type of infection which tends to occur in the elderly diabetic patient.[4] It results in unremitting pain, purulent discharge, and tends to invade cartilage, bone, nerve, and the adjacent soft tissues." Not only did he define the classic history and physical examination findings, he also was the first to describe the route of spread via the fissures of Santorini to the parotid gland and soft tissues in the neck and skull base. In his series, 12/13 had diabetes, 13/13 were caused by pseudomonas, 3/13 were bilateral, 6/13 had facial paralysis and 6/13 died of disease. Chandler advocated for aggressive surgical resection, given the lack of adequate anti-pseudomonal antibiotics at the time.[4] Over the past 50 years it has been shown that any condition that leads to an immunocompromised state, in addition to diabetes, has the potential to lead to SBO. It can occur in both children and adults, although the outcome in children appears more optimistic.[15,16] Aggressive surgical procedures have been abandoned for the most part, given advances in antibiotics, and lack of demonstrable benefit.[17,18]

SBO must be differentiated from chronic otitis externa, in which the ear canal demonstrates variable thickening of the skin with a resultant narrowing of the lumen. Senturia was the first to describe this entity with its pathologic correlation.[19] The primary symptom is itching, and the physical examination reveals excessive, dry adherent, exfoliated debris; mucopurulent drainage may also be found, with papules and foul odor.[19] Culture results often demonstrate gram-negative bacilli, but they vary considerably due to the widespread use of topical antibiotics.[20] Treatment is directed toward frequent cleaning and the use of acidifying agents. Surgery is rarely indicated but useful if canal narrowing leads to further complications.

PATIENT FACTORS PREDISPOSING TO SKULL BASE OSTEOMYELITIS AND PROGRESSION

The most frequently described risk factor for developing SBO is diabetes mellitus which is reported in 80% to 90% of cases.[21,22] Patients with SBO and diabetes often have worse outcomes including prolonged hospitalization and greater disease-specific mortality in comparison to non-diabetics.[23,24] In diabetics, the ear canal can be affected by microangiopathy and neuropathy predisposing to soft tissue infection with contiguous extension to the cranial base and potential for vascular involvement with hematogenous seeding. In this setting, antibiotic activity is reduced due to compromised microvascular perfusion.[25] Additionally, impairment of chemotaxis and phagocytosis of leukocytes and a higher cerumen pH foster bacterial overgrowth.[22,23] Pseudomonas aeruginosa, commonly identified in SBO, is an opportunistic pathogen that infects damaged or unhealthy tissues in patients with diabetes and is associated with virulence factors and biofilm formation.[26] While the duration of diabetes and poor blood sugar control have not correlated with SBO severity in all series, chronic hyperglycemia is known to drive angiopathy; and elevated hemoglobin A1c is associated with risk for limb loss in diabetic foot infection, underscoring the importance of glycemic management in diabetes-related infections including SBO.[25,26]

Advanced age, immunosuppression from uncontrolled Human Immunodeficiency Virus (HIV), organ transplantation, hematologic disorders, chemotherapy, and co-morbidities affecting the vascularization and oxygenation of bone have also been associated with SBO.[22,27] Age greater than 65 years portends worse SBO outcomes in some series with a greater need for surgical intervention.[21,23,27] Co-morbid conditions are found more frequently in older patients, while aging is also associated with significant shifts in the distribution and function of immune cells leading to loss of adaptive immunity and susceptibility to infection. As in diabetes, aging also impairs microvascular circulation.[28] SBO in patients with HIV is associated with low CD4 T lymphocyte counts (<100 cells/mm3) with pathogens other than Pseudomonas reported including Aspergillus spp. arising from a middle ear or mastoid source.[29,30] SBO is also occasionally reported in patients without underlying diabetes or immunosuppressive conditions with more favorable outcomes, reinforcing the need to maintain a high index of suspicion for SBO in any patient with extended otologic symptoms.[22]

DISEASE PRESENTATION

The hallmark presenting symptom of SBO is otalgia, typically described as a persistent and severe deep pain with nocturnal worsening. Pain can often be out of proportion to the findings on physical exam. Purulent foul-smelling drainage is present in most cases. Conductive hearing loss can occur when the ear canal becomes obstructed by drainage, edema, or granulation tissue.[27,31,32] On physical exam patients will commonly present with ear canal edema, purulent drainage, and characteristic granulation tissue at the bony cartilaginous junction of the ear canal. Tympanic membrane (TM) and middle ear are often uninvolved. However, the visualization of the TM is often obscured due to the ear canal edema[27,31,32].

Early presentation of SBO has significant overlap with acute or chronic otitis externa. Therefore, making the SBO diagnosis requires a high index of clinical suspicion in patient with known risk factors. Although some patients initially present with signs and symptoms to prompt further SBO workup, others are diagnosed when there is a lack of or incomplete response to otitis externa treatment.[32] In later stages, patients can develop additional symptoms indicating the spread of infection outside the confines of the ear canal in multiple directions through adjacent bone, soft tissue, or vascular extension.[33] Temporomandibular joint pain, swelling, and trismus occur with anterior spread through the fissures of Santorini. Facial nerve paralysis can develop with spread to the stylomastoid foramen, which can happen relatively early in the disease course compared to other cranial neuropathies.[34] Dysfunction of cranial nerves IX, X, XI can result from medial spread to the Jugular foramen resulting in dysphagia, dysphonia, aspiration, palatal and shoulder weakness.[35] More rarely, further spread to the petrous apex can result in deficits of cranial nerves II, III, V, VI resulting in vison changes, facial numbness, and double vison.[35,36] Contralateral symptoms can occur as infection spreads along the skull base.[33] Due to potential cranial nerve involvement, complete cranial nerve exam is important when SBO is suspected. Flexible laryngoscopy should be performed in patients with a concern of CN X dysfunction to aid in prompt diagnosis and treatment of aspiration.

Intracranial spread can result in cerebral venous thrombosis, meningitis, intracranial abscess.[33] Patients with intracranial complications may present with nausea, vomiting, headaches, and mental status change. Patients can present with areas of fluctuance indicating abscess formation in the surrounding extracranial soft tissues (neck, parotid, infratemporal fossa).[27,32] Importantly, SBO can also present without ear canal involvement. For this entity, the typical presentation consists of headaches that progress to cranial neuropathies when the infection is centered on the sphenoid or occipital bone.[37]

LABORATORY WORK-UP

Labs can be helpful in making the diagnosis of SBO and as markers of treatment response. Diabetes mellitus-related tests (blood glucose, hemoglobin A1C) should be obtained to determine glucose control in patients with the established diagnosis of diabetes or to check for new diagnoses.[38–40] Complete Blood Count (CBC) will typically be normal to slightly elevated.[27] Inflammatory markers such as erythrocyte sedimentation rate (ESR) and C-Reactive Protein (CRP) are typically elevated and can be used to monitor treatment response.[40,41]

Culture from ear drainage or tissue should be performed to guide treatment. *Pseudomonas aeruginosa* is found in the majority of patients.[27,42] *Aspergillus fumigatus* and *Candida spp* are the most common fungal organisms found with fungal infections being more common with immunosuppression.[27,43]

Tissue biopsy should be obtained to rule out malignancy given a significant overlap between the clinical and imaging characteristics of the two. Re-culture may also be necessary if the initial culture is negative or with poor response to antibiotic treatment.[44] Differential diagnosis to consider and differentiating factors are listed in **Table 1**.

Table 1
Differential diagnosis and differentiating factor

Differential Diagnosis	Differentiating Factors
Otitis Externa without osteomyelitis	• Lack of imaging findings supporting SBO • Resolution of symptoms with the short treatment of antibiotic/antifungal
Malignant Lesion of External Ear Canal or Nasopharynx	• Biopsy should be performed in all cases due to overall in clinical/imaging characteristics • Biopsy shows evidence of malignant disease
Cholesteatoma w/wo secondary infection	• Prior history of chronic ear disease • Clinical findings of cholesteatoma (retraction pocket, keratin debris, white middle ear mass, conductive hearing loss, and so forth). • Imaging features on CT (scutal erosion, ossicular involvement), MRI (restricted-diffusion on non-echo planar DWI)
Granulomatous disease	• Biopsy findings • Other sites of involvement

IMAGING

Diagnosis of SBO is challenging both clinically and on imaging, thus requiring a high degree of suspicion.[45] Imaging plays a central role not only in establishing accurate diagnosis, but also in evaluating for complications and guiding management. The imaging techniques commonly employed to diagnose SBO include noncontrast and contrast-enhanced CT, contrast-enhanced MRI, and nuclear imaging.[45–48]

CT is almost always performed as the first-line imaging method. High-resolution thin-section CT using a bone algorithm can easily be reformatted in multiple planes and is excellent to detect cortical bone erosions or trabecular bone destruction that accompany SBO.[45,47] It identifies the opacification of temporal bone structures, mucosal disease, and air-fluid levels in the paranasal sinuses and mastoid air cells.[45,47] Contrast-enhanced CT in soft tissue algorithm is useful to assess for cellulitis and soft-tissue infiltration, phlegmonous changes underneath the skull base, in the infratemporal region and rim enhancing abscess in the pre-clival soft tissues or along the mastoid tip. CT angiography or venography is employed to evaluate for vascular complications such as dural sinus or cavernous sinus thrombosis and neurovascular complications which are more common in aggressive fungal SBO.[45,47–49]

MRI is superior to CT for determining the complete extent of the disease process and is better in assessing bone marrow involvement and extraosseous soft tissue structures (**Fig. 1**A, B, D). A dedicated skull base MRI protocol (**Box 1**) is necessary for complete evaluation, including DWI, fat suppression, and thin section contrast-enhanced images. Early findings of SBO include nonspecific soft tissue thickening and enhancement in the EAC, with erosion at the petrotympanic fissure, obliteration of the retrocondylar fat pad, and with marked edema and inflammation of the periauricular soft tissues.[49] With progression, the soft tissue infection can spread via fascial planes to surrounding soft tissues and osseous structures and may extend to the skull base foramina to involve the cranial nerves and the intracranial compartment.[49] With advanced cases of SBO, bone marrow may become necrotic and form an abscess,

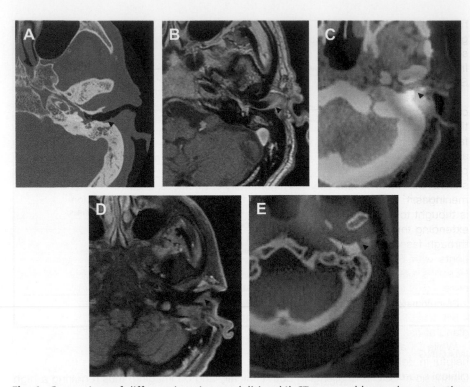

Fig. 1. Comparison of different imaging modalities. (*A*) CT temporal bone: demonstrating increased soft tissue and edema of left EAC, middle ear/mastoid opacification (*B*) MRI axial T1 w Gadolinium contrast with soft tissue enhancement along left EAC (*arrow*) (*C*) Follow-up Nuclear Medicine Gallium Fused SPECT CT scan shows marked tracer accumulation in left EAC (*arrow*) (*D*) MRI T1 w Gadolinium contrast shows the resolution of enhancement. (*E*) Nuclear Medicine Gallium Fused SPECT CT scan shows resolution of previously seen tracer accumulation (*arrow*).

with peripheral rim enhancement and central diffusion restriction. The soft-tissue abnormality in the nasopharynx may be the most prominent finding and therefore these cases are often misdiagnosed as infiltrative neoplasm, especially nasopharyngeal carcinoma.[50,51] Diffusion imaging also allows distinction between SBO and other

---

Box 1
MRI protocol for SBO

MRI PROTOCOL FOR SUSPECTED SKULL BASE OSTEOMYELITIS
   3-plane localizer
   Sagittal T1 3D
   Axial DWI (preferably readout-segmented echo-planar diffusion - rs-DWI)
   Axial T2 fat saturated 3 mm (preferably whole brain)
   Coronal STIR 3 mm
   Axial T1 3 mm
   Coronal T1 3 mm
   Postcontrast axial T1 3 mm with fat saturation
   Postcontrast coronal T1 3 mm with fat saturation
   Optional: MR Angiography or MR Venography (as necessary)

neoplastic mimics. Apparent diffusion coefficient (ADC) values in bacterial SBO are generally higher than those in nasopharyngeal carcinoma or lymphoma.[45,47,50] The soft-tissue invasion and neurovascular complications can occur before or without frank bone destruction, especially in early or aggressive diseases such as fungal SBO.[45]

SBO is generally categorized according to an anterior, posterior, medial, or an intracranial spreading pattern or a combination of these. In an *anterior* spreading pattern, the temporomandibular joint (TMJ), masticator space, parotid gland, or surrounding fat planes are involved. The *posterior* spreading pattern affects the mastoid process, and the *medial* spreading pattern affects the sphenoid, clivus, nasopharyngeal or pharyngeal muscles/fat, and cranial nerves IX, X, and XI. The *intracranial* pattern shows the involvement of the jugular fossa, jugular vein, sigmoid sinus, and meninges.[52] The spread of SBO from the external ear canal to the anterior pattern is thought to occur via the fissures of Santorini (which are not seen on imaging), by extending through osseocartilaginous junctions of the external ear canal, spreading through fascial planes and blood vessels to surrounding compartments. Some patients with SBO have a variant anatomic structure called a *persistent foramen of Huschke* aka, "foramen tympanicum," which is a dehiscence antero-inferiorly in the osseous external auditory canal (EAC) posterior-medial to the temporomandibular joint (TMJ). Its prevalence is higher in women and on the left side, and ranges from 4.6% to 20%. This anatomic pathway puts the TMJ, masticator space, and parotid gland at risk.

While CT and MRI are critical in the initial diagnosis of SBO, they are not necessarily helpful in determining real-time disease resolution as imaging findings generally lag clinical improvement. There can be improvement in soft-tissue findings which is likely the best imaging marker for improvement and response to treatment; but abnormalities of bone may persist for weeks to months despite adequate clinical response.[45] A variety of nuclear medicine studies are very sensitive in providing functional and metabolic information, and can help to confirm and localize infection to the skull base. These nuclear medicine studies are complementary to CT and MRI studies in monitoring treatment response. Technetium methylene diphosphonate (Tc99m MDP) bone scan, gallium-67 citrate (Ga-67) scan, and technetium-labeled white blood cell scan have all been used in patients with SBO but generally, the literature has variable data regarding the overall diagnostic value of these nuclear medicine tests with poor specificity. We, therefore, *advise against the routine use of these studies* in diagnosis or even follow-up of patients with SBO.[53] However, these examinations can serve as adjuncts in complicated patients with an unclear diagnosis and disease course (**Fig. 1**C, E). (18F) Fluorodeoxyglucose (FDG)-positron emission tomography (PET) CT has advantages over other nuclear studies with much wider availability, shorter imaging time, and higher spatial resolution and can be complementary to determine the extent of infection in confirmed cases of SBO and for the evaluation of treatment response.[54] Hybrid PET-MRI scanners offer exquisite soft-tissue detail and metabolic information in a single study. The summary of imaging teaching points is listed in **Box 2**.

SURGICAL MANAGEMENT

Tissue biopsy is required to confirm the diagnosis, to eliminate other possibilities such as cancer, and to determine the causative organisms. In the chronic draining ear, biopsy of any abnormal tissue in the ear canal is easily performed in the outpatient clinic under the operative microscope using cup forceps. Ear polyps can be removed and

---

Box 2
Imaging pearls

- Enhancement and fullness without destruction of fascial planes and absence of a discrete soft tissue mass may support a diagnosis of SBO over tumor.
- early changes of SBO are subtle and easily missed. One of the earliest findings is infiltration of the retrocondylar fat pad.
- Soft-tissue infiltration of the retroantral fat and pterygopalatine fossa with obliteration of normal fat in these regions is typical of SBO associated with invasive sinusitis.
- knowledge of persistent foramen of Huschke is important to identify patients with early SBO and its patterns of extension, thus aiding in improved diagnosis and outcomes.

---

sent for culture. These types of biopsies do not always reveal the causative organism. Deeper biopsy material can be obtained through either image-guided biopsy or surgery. CT-guided biopsy can often be performed and is a less invasive procedure than open biopsy.[55] For infections that originate in the central skull base, endoscopic endonasal approach can be used to obtain appropriate biopsy and culture material.[56] For infections that arise from the middle ear and mastoid, mastoidectomy can yield appropriate tissue. Indications for mastoidectomy are listed in **Box 3**.

Since the infection is diffuse, mastoidectomy is not curative for this illness.[18] The goal of mastoidectomy is limited to obtaining appropriate tissue for culture and pathologic examination, and not the restoration of hearing (see **Box 3**).[17,42] Myringotomy and tube can be considered to allow drainage of the middle ear. Mastoidectomy is generally limited to abscess drainage, but sigmoid sinus thrombectomy can be performed when signs of Lemierre's syndrome are present.[57]

For central SBO, where the infection is in the clivus and petrous apex, a targeted approach via an extended nasopharyngeal biopsy can be helpful to obtain tissue to pathologic diagnosis and microbiology culture.[56] Any purulent material can be gathered on swabs for culture. Thickened mucosa and granulation tissue should be sent for pathologic examination and culture. Since the underlying infection is bony, sending bone specimens obtained with curettes or rongeurs can be helpful at identifying the offending organism.

In a systematic review of surgery for SBO, Mahdyoun and colleagues identified 21 publications covering 439 patients, and the majority of authors described limited surgery to remove bone sequestrate from the EAC or to obtain histologic and

---

Box 3
Surgery indications

Mastoidectomy Indications
  Clinical Evidence of Middle Ear/Mastoid Cavity disease
  Lack of Confirmed Diagnosis
  Lack of Causative Micro-organism
  Radiographic Evidence of Mastoid Involvement
  Inappropriateness or Unavailability of Less Invasive Technique for biopsy or diagnosis (ie, image-guided biopsy)
  Lack of Response to Medical Therapy
  Drainage of Abscess
  Debridement of Necrotic Tissue
  Possibly Facial Nerve Decompression for Facial Paralysis

microbiologic samples.[58] Stevens and colleagues performed a systematic review of the literature to determine criteria for separating malignant otitis externa (MOE) into severe cases, where surgery might be necessary, and nonsevere cases, where no surgery is required.[59] They identified four clinical variables (facial nerve palsy, disease relapse, required surgery, positive fungal culture) and 5 radiologic variables (TMJ, Infratemporal fossa, or tegmen erosion, and nasopharyngeal or intracranial involvement). In their article, severe cases demonstrated at least one of the following characteristics: (1) facial palsy, (2) two or more clinical variables other than facial palsy,[60] two or more radiographic variables, (4) one or more clinical variables and one or more radiographic variable. Although 12 out of 28 patients met their criteria for severe disease, only 2 patients underwent surgery.

Peled and colleagues described a relatively large series of 20 patients who underwent surgery out of a series of 83 patients with necrotizing otitis externa.[61] Their series consisted of local debridement (n = 7), canal wall up mastoidectomy (CWU) (n = 4), canal wall down (CWD) mastoidectomy (n = 7) and CWD with facial nerve decompression (n = 2). The primary indication for surgery was a lack of response to prolonged antibiotic therapy, and this indication covered 90% of their surgical patients. Lack of response was determined based on pain control, general condition, and physical findings after 2 weeks of antibiotic therapy. All surgical patients had evidence of extensive temporal bone involvement on high-resolution temporal bone CT. Their previous work indicated that elderly patients (average age 77 years) were at higher risk for conservative treatment failure and more likely to require surgery.[21] Others have used a 3-week,[62,63] 4-week,[64,65] or 6-week[23] treatment duration without improvement to consider the case refractory. Shavit and colleagues reported on 88 patients with SBO, of which 20 (23%) had a surgical procedure.[66] They performed external canal debridement in 12 and mastoidectomy in 8 (CWU in 4, CWD in 4).

A special consideration is made for patients with progressive facial weakness in the setting of SBO. Unlike the lower cranial nerves (CN IX-XII), facial paralysis in the setting of SBO generally does not improve with medical management alone.[35] Unlike Bell's palsy, where the facial nerve is compromised at the labyrinthine segment due to viral-induced swelling, facial nerve paralysis in SBO might be diffuse and related to granulation tissue and toxins along its course causing impaired axonal conduction.[35] Freeman and colleagues reported on 14 patients with facial paralysis and SBO and compared the facial nerve outcomes between patients who underwent surgical decompression versus those that were observed.[67] None of the patients treated with medical management had any significant improvement in facial function. Of the patients treated with mastoidectomy and facial nerve decompression, 3 of 5 patients had significant improvement (defined as a decrease of at least 2 points on House-Brackmann facial nerve scale.[68] In the mastoidectomy only group, 2 of 5 patients experienced a significant improvement on the HB scale. However, statistical analysis demonstrated no significant difference across the three cohorts, given the small numbers in the study. Patients who experienced the greatest improvement in facial function had facial nerve decompression <14 days from the onset of paralysis, a finding very similar to what is seen in Bell's palsy patients.[69] The goal of facial nerve decompression within 14 days can be difficult to achieve in a disease that can take weeks to manifest and be diagnosed.

Peleg and colleagues reported 18 patients with SBO, of which 5 had severe disease.[64] These 5 patients underwent extensive operations, including any combination of radical mastoidectomy, temporomandibular joint (TMJ) excision, parotidectomy, partial removal of the zygomatic arch, and bony/soft tissue debridement of the infratemporal fossa and skull base; however, they did not report any outcomes. Omran and colleagues performed similar extensive surgery (radical mastoidectomy, TMJ excision, partial removal of the zygomatic arch and debridement of the occipital bone and skull base).[70] Out of 10 patients with recurrent disease, 2 patients died, and 2 patients deteriorated during follow-up. Yigider and colleagues performed surgery in 9 out of 26 patients with SBO.[71] Five patients had radical mastoidectomy and 4 had subtotal petrosectomy. Two patients who underwent surgical intervention died of disease. Visosky and colleagues described a circumferential petrosectomy for patients that fail to improve with medical management or patients with impending complications.[72] These patients presented with complex CN deficits, such as Tolosa-Hunt syndrome or Gradenigo syndrome, and substantial inflammation around the petrous and cavernous carotid artery. In their procedure, most of the temporal bone was removed via combined retrolabyrinthine-apical petrosectomy and fallopian bridge technique. Middle fossa craniotomy is performed for petrosectomy. Their report describes 5 cases with disease resolution in all patients. Some authors have used tympanomastoid surgery after 6 months of treatment for removing the inflammatory lesion as much as possible.[73]

MICROBIOLOGY AND MEDICAL TREATMENT

Once the diagnosis of SBO is established, baseline cultures should be obtained whenever possible prior to initiating antimicrobial treatment. The culture data can be valuable when treatment fails or drug toxicities emerge. While *Pseudomonas aeruginosa* remains the most common organism seen in SBO,[21] other organisms such as *Staphylococcus aureus* (either methicillin sensitive or resistant) and other Gram-negative rods can also cause SBO. This fact further supports the importance of obtaining cultures prior to initiating empiric anti-Pseudomonal therapy.

Culture results should be examined critically in particular when they yield organisms which are unlikely to be pathogenic and may be colonizing the ear canal superficially such as coagulase-negative Staphylococci or Enterococci. Moreover, topical antimicrobial and antiseptic therapies that patients have received prior to evaluation and diagnosis may decrease the yield of true pathogen growth in culture.[74] Decisions on whether to treat potentially non-pathogenic organisms (ie, coagulase-negative Staphylococci or Enterococci) when they are the only organisms that grow in culture can be challenging. The decision to treat non-pathogenic organisms, in addition to empirically treating Pseudomonas (and other Gram-negative rods), is individualized depending on the patient's degree of immunocompromise and severity of disease. Since Pseudomonas is the most common SBO pathogen, treatment regimen that includes anti-Pseudomonal therapy is reasonable when no other pathogenic organism is found. It is critical to monitor these patients closely with close surveillance and ongoing consideration of alternative pathogens such as fungi in refractory cases.

The quinolones (ciprofloxacin and levofloxacin) are the only oral anti-Pseudomonal agents available to treat systemic infection. Due to their high oral bioavailability and bone penetration, these drugs are first-line treatment options for presumed or confirmed susceptible Pseudomonal infections. High "anti-Pseudomonal" dosing is appropriate (750 mg po BID for ciprofloxacin and 750 mg po daily for levofloxacin) with dose adjustment for renal insufficiency. When a Pseudomonal isolate is grown that is quinolone resistant or when the patient cannot tolerate quinolones, intravenous anti-Pseudomonal options include cephalosporins (cefepime or ceftazidime) or beta-lactam/beta-lactamase inhibitor piperacillin-tazobactam. These medications are favored over carbapenems (imipenem and meropenem) when possible, because Pseudomonas spp have the ability to develop resistance to carbapenems quickly when a high organism burden is present, and because they can be used as monother-apy without an additional agent. In severe cases, carbapenems can be given in com-bination with a quinolone. In cases where a highly resistant Pseudomonas is cultured, the use of newer generation cephalosporins (eg, cefiderocol) or treating with combina-tions of agents may be necessary. While aminoglycosides are active against Pseudo-monas, given their potential nephrotoxicity and ototoxicity with prolonged use, they are not ideal first-line therapy for SBO.

Fungal pathogens which are more common in diabetics and other immunocompro-mised hosts, can plan a role in SBO, potentially being a culprit in "culture negative" cases potentially due to the difficulty in culturing fungi from clinical samples.[63] Asper-gillus is the fungus most commonly seen in progressive SBO though other mold have been described rarely.[75] When Aspergillus is suspected based on exam concerning for mold or angioinvasion, or there is ongoing disease progression despite being on broad antibacterial therapy, antifungal therapy is appropriate with tissue debridement as needed. Voriconazole has high oral bioavailability and would generally be first-line anti-fungal therapy for Aspergillus. If drug interactions or intolerability preclude its use, other options now include oral isovuconazole or posaconazole, intravenous echino-candins and intravenous liposomal amphotericin B. Summary of treatment paradigm is shown in **Fig. 2**.

The specific duration of antimicrobial therapy in SBO cannot be predetermined dogmatically. As is the case for most infections involving bone, at least 6 weeks of sys-temic antimicrobials are indicated with ongoing close clinical follow up to determine if disease progression has halted, stabilized, and then improved. At times with extensive disease, treatment response can be slow and extended antibiotic regimens may be appropriate. Ongoing monitoring for patient adherence, drug tolerability, and toxicity should also continue concomitantly. When inflammatory markers such as ESR and CRP are highly elevated at the time of diagnosis, periodic monitoring of these markers while on therapy (eg, every 2–3 weeks) can be an adjunct measure in determining treatment duration. However, these lab results are notoriously non-specific and can

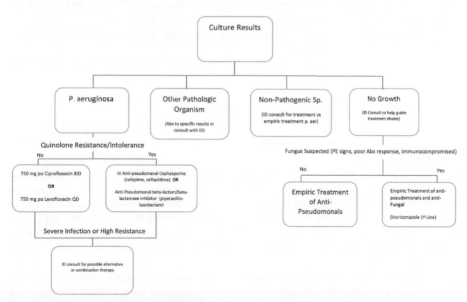

Fig. 2. Medical treatment algorithm.

at times be unhelpful. If the patient has improved on antimicrobials, the decision to stop treatment should be team-based approached, using interval clinical course and imaging studies. Follow-up for relapse should be continued in the year following discontinuation.

SUMMARY

SBO is a life-threatening disease that requires a high index of suspicion based on these patients complex underlying medical co-morbidities and clinician's acumen. Once a diagnosis is made, is it critical to communicate and work closely with other multidisciplinary teams (neuroradiology for appropriate choice of imaging study and interpretation; infectious disease for appropriate medical treatment and duration; internist to properly manage their underlying medical co-morbidities). Though this disease has been around for centuries with many different names, SBO is a chronic bone infection with high morbidity and mortality. Despite advances in imaging, the diagnosis is first made based on clinical judgment, appropriate culture, and tissue biopsy. Appropriate duration of medical treatment is crucial to avoid incomplete treatment that result in relapse and complications.

REFERENCES

1. Brunner H. Pathologic Changes of Temporal Bone in Osteomyelitis of Skull. Laryngoscope 1942;52:954–67.
2. Kelemen G., Osteomyelitis of the Temporal Bone. *Otolaryngology*, H.P.S. G.M. Coates, and M.V. Miller. editors. 1955: Hagerstown, MD, 26.
3. Meltzer PEM, Kelemen G. Pyocyaneous Osteomyelitis of the Temporal Bone, Mandible and Zygoma. Laryngoscope 1959;69:1300–16.
4. Chandler JR. Malignant external otitis. Laryngoscope 1968;78(8):1257–94.
5. Nadol JB Jr. Histopathology of Pseudomonas osteomyelitis of the temporal bone starting as malignant external otitis. Am J Otolaryngol 1980;1(5):359–71.
6. Kohut RI, Lindsay JR. Necrotizing ("malignant") external otitis histopathologic processes. Ann Otol Rhinol Laryngol 1979;88(5 Pt 1):714–20.
7. Toulmouche MA. Observations d'Otorrhee Cerebrale: Suivis des Reflexions. Gaz. Med. De Paris 1838;6:422–6.
8. Zaufal E. Ueber das Vorkommen blauer Otorrhoen. Arch f Ohrenheilk 1873;6(2): 207–18.
9. Chambers TR. Bacteriological Examinations of Otitis Media Purulenta and Suppurative Mastoiditis. A.M.A 1900;35:1405–7.
10. Wakefield A. Report of Fatal Case of Latent Temporo-sphenoidal Abscess of Otitic Origin Followed by Multiple Secondary Cerebral Abscesses. Arch Otol 1904;33:273–82.
11. Voss, O., Der Bacillus pyocyaneus im Ohr. Veroeff. a d Geb.d Militaer-Sanitaetswesens, 1906. 33:34: p. 1197.
12. Haymann L. Experimentelle Studien zur Pathologie der akutentzuendlichen Prozesse im Mittelohr (und im Labyrinth). Arch. F Ohrenheik 1914;95:98–144.
13. Wirth E. Subakute Mastoiditis durch Mischinfektionen von Bacillus pyocanaeus und Streptococcus anhaemolyticus. Zeitschr. f Hals-Nasen-Ohrenheilk 1926; 17(2):188–91.
14. Brunner, H., Intracranial Complications of Ear, Nose and Throat Infections. 1946.
15. Sobie S, Brodsky L, Stanievich JF. Necrotizing external otitis in children: report of two cases and review of the literature. Laryngoscope 1987;97(5):598–601.

16. Castro R, Robinson N, Klein J, Geimeier W. Malignant external otitis and mastoiditis associated with an IgG4 subclass deficiency in a child. Del Med J 1990; 62(12):1417–21.

17. Stapleton E, Watson G. Emerging themes in necrotising otitis externa: a scoping review of the literature 2011-2020 and recommendations for future research. J Laryngol Otol 2021;1–30.

18. Nguyen PT, Chang J, Shahlaie K, et al. Skull base infections, their complications, and management. NeuroRadiol J 2023. https://doi.org/10.1177/19714009221140540. 19714009221140540.

19. Senturia BH. What's new in the treatment of otitis externa: the otologist's viewpoint. Trans Am Acad Ophthalmol Otolaryngol 1957;61(3):347–59.

20. Bojrab DI, Bruderly T, Abdulrazzak Y. Otitis externa. Otolaryngol Clin North Am 1996;29(5):761–82.

21. Peled C, El-Seid S, Bahat-Dinur A, et al. Necrotizing Otitis Externa-Analysis of 83 Cases: Clinical Findings and Course of Disease. Otol Neurotol 2019;40(1):56–62.

22. Chen JC, Yeh C, Shiao A, et al. Temporal bone osteomyelitis: the relationship with malignant otitis externa, the diagnostic dilemma, and changing trends. Sci World J 2014;2014:591714.

23. Trevino Gonzalez JL, Reyes Suarez LL, Hernandez de Leon JE. Malignant otitis externa: An updated review. Am J Otolaryngol 2021;42(2):102894.

24. Sideris G, Latzonis J, Avgeri C, et al. A Different Era for Malignant Otitis Externa: The Non-Diabetic and Non-Immunocompromised Patients. J Int Adv Otol 2022; 18(1):20–4.

25. Forbes JM, Cooper MF. Mechanisms of diabetic complications. Physiol Rev 2013;93(1):137–88.

26. Morin CD, Déziel E, Gauthier J, et al. An Organ System-Based Synopsis of Pseudomonas aeruginosa Virulence. Virulence 2021;12(1):1469–507.

27. Carfrae MJ, Kesser BW. Malignant otitis externa. Otolaryngol Clin North Am 2008; 41(3):537–49, viii-ix.

28. Weyand CM, Goronzy JJ. Aging of the Immune System. Mechanisms and Therapeutic Targets. Ann Am Thorac Soc 2016;13(Suppl 5):S422–8.

29. Carney AS. Malignant otitis externa. Scott-Brown's Otorhinolaryngol Head Neck Surg 2008;3:3336–41.

30. Hern JD, Almeyda J, Thomas D, et al. Malignant otitis externa in HIV and AIDS. J Laryngol Otol 1996;110(8):770–5.

31. Cohen D, Friedman P. The diagnostic criteria of malignant external otitis. J Laryngol Otol 1987;101(3):216–21.

32. Sharma S, Corrah T, Singh A. Management of Necrotizing Otitis Externa: Our Experience with Forty-Three Patients. J Int Adv Otol 2017;13(3):394–8.

33. Kwon BJ, Han M, Oh S, et al. MRI findings and spreading patterns of necrotizing external otitis: is a poor outcome predictable? Clin Radiol 2006;61(6):495–504.

34. Soudry E, Joshua BZ, Sulkes J, Nageris BI. Characteristics and prognosis of malignant external otitis with facial paralysis. Arch Otolaryngol Head Neck Surg 2007;133(10):1002–4.

35. Mani N, Sudhoff H, Rajagopal S, et al. Cranial nerve involvement in malignant external otitis: implications for clinical outcome. Laryngoscope 2007;117(5): 907–10.

36. Patel B, Souqiyyeh A, Ali A. A Case of Transient, Isolated Cranial Nerve VI Palsy due to Skull Base Osteomyelitis. Case Rep Infect Dis 2014;2014:369867.

37. Chang PC, Fischbein NJ, Holliday RA. Central skull base osteomyelitis in patients without otitis externa: imaging findings. AJNR Am J Neuroradiol 2003;24(7): 1310–6.

38. Lee SK, Lee SA, Seon SW, et al. Analysis of Prognostic Factors in Malignant External Otitis. Clin Exp Otorhinolaryngol 2017;10(3):228–35.

39. Marina S, Goutham MK, Rajeshwary A, et al. A retrospective review of 14 cases of malignant otitis externa. J Otol 2019;14(2):63–6.

40. Kaya İ, Sezgin B, Eraslan S, et al. Malignant Otitis Externa: A Retrospective Analysis and Treatment Outcomes. Turk Arch Otorhinolaryngol 2018;56(2):106–10.

41. Faizal B, Surendran B, Kumar M. Comparative study of reliability of inflammatory markers over 18-FDG-PET CT scan in monitoring skull base osteomyelitis. Braz J Otorhinolaryngol 2022;88(5):691–700.

42. Rubin Grandis J, Branstetter BFt, Yu VL. The changing face of malignant (necrotising) external otitis: clinical, radiological, and anatomic correlations. Lancet Infect Dis 2004;4(1):34–9.

43. Mion M, Bovo R, Marchese-Ragona R, Martini A. Outcome predictors of treatment effectiveness for fungal malignant external otitis: a systematic review. Acta Otorhinolaryngol Ital 2015;35(5):307–13.

44. Bernstein JM, Holland NJ, Porter GC, Maw AR. Resistance of Pseudomonas to ciprofloxacin: implications for the treatment of malignant otitis externa. J Laryngol Otol 2007;121(2):118–23.

45. Chapman PR, Choudhary G, Singhal A. Skull Base Osteomyelitis: A Comprehensive Imaging Review. AJNR Am J Neuroradiol 2021;42(3):404–13.

46. Takata J, Hopkins M, Alexander V, et al. Systematic review of the diagnosis and management of necrotising otitis externa: Highlighting the need for high-quality research. Clin Otolaryngol 2023;48(3):381–94.

47. Álvarez Jáñez F, Barriga LQ, Iñigo TR, Roldán Lora F. Diagnosis of Skull Base Osteomyelitis. Radiographics 2021;41(1):156–74.

48. Hegde AN, Mohan S, Pandya A, et al. Imaging in infections of the head and neck. Neuroimaging Clin N Am 2012;22(4):727–54.

49. Mohan S, Hoeffner E, Bigelow D, et al. Applications of magnetic resonance imaging in adult temporal bone disorders. Magn Reson Imaging Clin N Am 2012; 20(3):545–72.

50. Ozgen B, Oguz KK, Cila A. Diffusion MR imaging features of skull base osteomyelitis compared with skull base malignancy. AJNR Am J Neuroradiol 2011;32(1): 179–84.

51. Baba A, Kurokawa R, Kurokawa M, et al. Dynamic Contrast-Enhanced MRI Parameters and Normalized ADC Values Could Aid Differentiation of Skull Base Osteomyelitis from Nasopharyngeal Cancer. AJNR Am J Neuroradiol 2023; 44(1):74–8.

52. van der Meer WL, van Tilburg M, Mitea C, Postma AA. A Persistent Foramen of Huschke: A Small Road to Misery in Necrotizing External Otitis. AJNR Am J Neuroradiol 2019;40(9):1552–6.

53. Moss WJ, Finegersh A, Narayanan A, Chan JYK. Meta-analysis does not support routine traditional nuclear medicine studies for malignant otitis. Laryngoscope 2020;130(7):1812–6.

54. Dondi F, Albano D, Treglia G, et al. Could [(18)F]FDG PET/CT or PET/MRI Be Useful in Patients with Skull Base Osteomyelitis? Diagnostics 2022;12(9).

55. Singhal A, Sotoudeh H, Chapman PR. Skull base osteomyelitis imaging. Curr Opin Otolaryngol Head Neck Surg 2021;29(5):333–41.

56. Thomas R. Targeted skull base biopsies in the management of central skull base osteomyelitis. Clin Otolaryngol 2021;46(1):72–4.
57. Thevis M, Leow T, Bekkers S, et al. Diagnosis, treatment and prognosis of otomastoiditis induced by Fusobacterium necrophorum: A retrospective multicentre cohort study. Anaerobe 2022;76:102587.
58. Mahdyoun P, Pulcini C, Gahide I, et al. Necrotizing otitis externa: a systematic review. Otol Neurotol 2013;34(4):620–9.
59. Stevens SM, Lambert P, Baker A, et al. Malignant otitis externa: a novel stratification protocol for predicting treatment outcomes. Otol Neurotol 2015;36(9): 1492–8.
60. Slattery WH 3rd, Brackmann DE. Skull base osteomyelitis. Malignant external otitis. Otolaryngol Clin North Am 1996;29(5):795–806.
61. Peled C, Parra A, El-Saied S, et al. Surgery for necrotizing otitis externa-indications and surgical findings. Eur Arch Otorhinolaryngol 2020;277(5):1327–34.
62. Joshua BZ, Sulkes J, Raveh E, et al. Predicting outcome of malignant external otitis. Otol Neurotol 2008;29(3):339–43.
63. Gruber M, Roitman A, Doweck I, et al. Clinical utility of a polymerase chain reaction assay in culture-negative necrotizing otitis externa. Otol Neurotol 2015;36(4): 733–6.
64. Peleg U, Perez R, Raveh D, et al. Stratification for malignant external otitis. Otolaryngol Head Neck Surg 2007;137(2):301–5.
65. Soudry E, Hamzany Y, Preis M, et al. Malignant external otitis: analysis of severe cases. Otolaryngology-Head Neck Surg (Tokyo) 2011;144(5):758–62.
66. Stern Shavit S, Soudry E, Hamzany Y, Nageris B. Malignant external otitis: Factors predicting patient outcomes. Am J Otolaryngol 2016;37(5):425–30.
67. Freeman MH, Perkins EL, Tawfik KO, et al. Facial Paralysis in Skull Base Osteomyelitis Comparison of Surgical and Nonsurgical Management. Laryngoscope 2023;133(1):179–83.
68. House JW, Brackmann DE. Facial nerve grading system. Otolaryngology-head and neck surgery 1985;93(2):146.
69. Gantz BJ, Rubinstein J, Gidley P, et al. Surgical management of Bell's palsy. Laryngoscope 1999;109(8):1177–88.
70. Omran AA, El Garem HF, Al Alem RK. Recurrent malignant otitis externa: management and outcome. Eur Arch Oto-Rhino-Laryngol 2012;269(3):807–11.
71. Yigider AP, Ovunc O, Arslan E, et al. Malignant Otitis Externa: How to Monitor the Disease in Outcome Estimation? Medeni Med J 2021;36(1):23–9.
72. Visosky AMB, Isaacson B, Oghalai JS. Circumferential petrosectomy for petrous apicitis and cranial base osteomyelitis. Otol Neurotol 2006;27(7):1003–13.
73. Takahashi K, Morita Y, Ogi M, et al. Optimal Diagnostic Criteria and a Staging System for Otogenic Skull Base Osteomyelitis. J Neurol Surg B Skull Base 2022;83(Suppl 2):e484–91.
74. Chaabouni MA, Achour I, Yousfi G, et al. Culture-negative necrotizing otitis externa: diagnosis and management. Egypt J Otolaryngol 2023;39:30.
75. Akhtar F, Iftikhar J, Azhar M, et al. Skull Base Osteomyelitis: A Single-Center Experience. Cureus 2021;13(12):e20162.

UNITED STATES POSTAL SERVICE ®
Statement of Ownership, Management, and Circulation
(All Periodicals Except Requester Publications)

1. Publication Title
OTOLARYNGOLOGIC CLINICS OF NORTH AMERICA

2. Publication Number
466 – 550

3. Filing Date
9/18/2023

4. Issue Frequency
FEB, APR, JUN, AUG, OCT, DEC

5. Number of Issues Published Annually
6

6. Annual Subscription Price
$468.00

7. Complete Mailing Address of Known Office of Publication (Not printer) (Street, city, county, state, and ZIP+4®)
ELSEVIER INC.
230 Park Avenue, Suite 800
New York, NY 10169

Contact Person: Malathi Samayan
Telephone (include area code): 91-44-4299 #507

8. Complete Mailing Address of Headquarters or General Business Office of Publisher (Not printer)
ELSEVIER INC.
230 Park Avenue, Suite 800
New York, NY 10169

9. Full Names and Complete Mailing Addresses of Publisher, Editor, and Managing Editor (Do not leave blank)

Publisher (Name and complete mailing address)
Dolores Meloni, ELSEVIER INC.
1600 JOHN F KENNEDY BLVD. SUITE 1600
PHILADELPHIA, PA 19103-2899

Editor (Name and complete mailing address)
Stacy Eastman, ELSEVIER INC.
1600 JOHN F KENNEDY BLVD. SUITE 1600
PHILADELPHIA, PA 19103-2899

Managing Editor (Name and complete mailing address)
PATRICK MANLEY, ELSEVIER INC.
1600 JOHN F KENNEDY BLVD. SUITE 1600
PHILADELPHIA, PA 19103-2899

10. Owner (Do not leave blank. If the publication is owned by a corporation, give the name and address of the corporation immediately followed by the names and addresses of all stockholders owning or holding 1 percent or more of the total amount of stock. If not owned by a corporation, give the names and addresses of the individual owners. If owned by a partnership or other unincorporated firm, give its name and address as well as those of each individual owner. If the publication is published by a nonprofit organization, give its name and address.)

Full Name	Complete Mailing Address
WHOLLY OWNED SUBSIDIARY OF REED/ELSEVIER, US HOLDINGS	1600 JOHN F KENNEDY BLVD. SUITE 1600 PHILADELPHIA, PA 19103-2899

11. Known Bondholders, Mortgagees, and Other Security Holders Owning or Holding 1 Percent or More of Total Amount of Bonds, Mortgages, or Other Securities. If none, check box. ► ☐ None

Full Name	Complete Mailing Address
N/A	

12. Tax Status (For completion by nonprofit organizations authorized to mail at nonprofit rates) (Check one)
The purpose, function, and nonprofit status of this organization and the exempt status for federal income tax purposes:
☒ Has Not Changed During Preceding 12 Months
☐ Has Changed During Preceding 12 Months (Publisher must submit explanation of change with this statement)

PS Form 3526, July 2014 (Page 1 of 4 (see instructions page 4)) PSN: 7530-01-000-9931 PRIVACY NOTICE: See our privacy policy on www.usps.com.

---

13. Publication Title
OTOLARYNGOLOGIC CLINICS OF NORTH AMERICA

14. Issue Date for Circulation Data Below
AUGUST 2023

15. Extent and Nature of Circulation

		Average No. Copies Each Issue During Preceding 12 Months	No. Copies of Single Issue Published Nearest to Filing Date
a. Total Number of Copies (Net press run)		189	185
b. Paid Circulation (By Mail and Outside the Mail)	(1) Mailed Outside-County Paid Subscriptions Stated on PS Form 3541 (Include paid distribution above nominal rate, advertiser's proof copies, and exchange copies)	102	102
	(2) Mailed In-County Paid Subscriptions Stated on PS Form 3541 (Include paid distribution above nominal rate, advertiser's proof copies, and exchange copies)	0	0
	(3) Paid Distribution Outside the Mails Including Sales Through Dealers and Carriers, Street Vendors, Counter Sales, and Other Paid Distribution Outside USPS®	62	56
	(4) Paid Distribution by Other Classes of Mail Through the USPS (e.g., First-Class Mail®)	22	24
c. Total Paid Distribution (Sum of 15b (1), (2), (3), and (4))	►	186	182
d. Free or Nominal Rate Distribution (By Mail and Outside the Mail)	(1) Free or Nominal Rate Outside-County Copies included on PS Form 3541	2	2
	(2) Free or Nominal Rate In-County Copies included on PS Form 3541	0	0
	(3) Free or Nominal Rate Copies Mailed at Other Classes Through the USPS (e.g., First-Class Mail)	0	0
	(4) Free or Nominal Rate Distribution Outside the Mail (Carriers or other means)	1	1
e. Total Free or Nominal Rate Distribution (Sum of 15d (1), (2), (3) and (4))	►	3	3
f. Total Distribution (Sum of 15c and 15e)	►	189	185
g. Copies not Distributed (See Instructions to Publishers #4 (page 43))	►	0	0
h. Total (Sum of 15f and g)	►	189	185
i. Percent Paid (15c divided by 15f times 100)		98.41%	98.38%

* If you are claiming electronic copies, go to line 16 on page 3. If you are not claiming electronic copies, skip to line 17 on page 3.

16. Electronic Copy Circulation

	Average No. Copies Each Issue During Preceding 12 Months	No. Copies of Single Issue Published Nearest to Filing Date
a. Paid Electronic Copies	►	
b. Total Paid Print Copies (Line 15c) + Paid Electronic Copies (Line 16a)	►	
c. Total Print Distribution (Line 15f) + Paid Electronic Copies (Line 16a)	►	
d. Percent Paid (Both Print & Electronic Copies) (16b divided by 16c × 100)	►	

☐ I certify that 50% of all my distributed copies (electronic and print) are paid above a nominal price.

17. Publication of Statement of Ownership
☒ If the publication is a general publication, publication of this statement is required. Will be printed in the October 2023 issue of this publication.
☐ Publication not required.

18. Signature and Title of Editor, Publisher, Business Manager, or Owner

Malathi Samayan
Malathi Samayan - Distribution Controller

Date: 9/18/2023

I certify that all information furnished on this form is true and complete. I understand that anyone who furnishes false or misleading information on this form or who omits material or information requested on the form may be subject to criminal sanctions (including fines and imprisonment) and/or civil sanctions (including civil penalties).

PS Form 3526, July 2014 (Page 3 of 4) PRIVACY NOTICE: See our privacy policy on www.usps.com

Moving?

Make sure your subscription moves with you!

To notify us of your new address, find your **Clinics Account Number** (located on your mailing label above your name), and contact customer service at:

Email: journalscustomerservice-usa@elsevier.com

800-654-2452 (subscribers in the U.S. & Canada)
314-447-8871 (subscribers outside of the U.S. & Canada)

Fax number: 314-447-8029

Elsevier Health Sciences Division
Subscription Customer Service
3251 Riverport Lane
Maryland Heights, MO 63043

*To ensure uninterrupted delivery of your subscription, please notify us at least 4 weeks in advance of move.

Printed and bound by CPI Group (UK) Ltd, Croydon, CR0 4YY

03/10/2024

01040468-0016